Monographs of the
American Association on Mental Retardation, 12

Michael J. Begab, Series Editor

The Treatment of Severe Behavior Disorders

Behavior Analysis Approaches

Edited by

Ennio Cipani
University
of the Pacific

The Treatment of Severe Behavior Disorders

Behavior Analysis Approaches

Published by
American Association on Mental Retardation
1719 Kalorama Road, NW
Washington, DC 20009   U.S.A.

The points of view herein are those of the authors and do not neccessarily represent the official policy or opinion of the American Association on Mental Retardation. Publication does not imply endorsement by the Editor, the Association, or its individual members.

No. 12, Monographs of the American Association on Mental Retardation (ISSN 0895-8009)

Library of Congress Cataloging-in-Publication Data

The Treatment of severe behavior disorders.

    (Monograph of the American Association on Mental Retardation, ISSN 0895-8009; 12)
    Includes bibliographies.
    1. Behavior disorders in children—Treatment. 2. Behavior therapy for children. I. Cipani, Ennio. II. Series. [DNLM: 1. Behavior Therapy. 2. Child Behavior Disorders—therapy. 3. Mental Retardation—rehabilitation. W1 M0559J no. 12 / WM 307.M5 T784]
RJ506.B44T74 1989   618.92′89142   89-6556
ISBN 0-940898-21-7 (pbk.)

Printed in the United States of America

Contents

Foreword

Norris G. Haring
University of Washington

Advances in the technology of behavior management are occurring at such an accelerated rate that it makes the review and discussion of these accomplishments especially compelling. Therefore, the American Association on Mental Retardation selection of this topic for a monograph to be included in its distinguished series of publications is very timely indeed.

Dr. Cipani's introduction provides a thorough overview of the purpose and content of this monograph, which is a major summary of the research undertaken during the past decade, especially the developments in behavior management during the most recent five years. Previously, the application of behavior principles with individuals who have severe behavior disorders concentrated on the systematic arrangement of events that are either antecedent to and/or a consequence of specific behaviors. The success we have experienced in the application of these principles has been exemplified in classrooms and clinics throughout the country.

The major work of the 1970s was Alan Kazdin's *History of Behavior Modification* (1978). This excellent, comprehensive volume reviewed and evaluated research findings and applications of behavior modification procedures, including developments during the late 1970s. Kazdin encompassed a variety of philosophical positions and assumptions about the causes of behavior, the interpretation of research results, and the appropriateness of intervention strategies. In contrast to Kazdin's book, the present volume is more precisely focused in regard to target population and the strategies of behavior intervention and management.

The Kazdin book marks progress starting with the now-classic *Journal of Applied Behavior Analysis* article, "Some Current Dimensions of Applied Behavior Analysis," by Baer, Wolf, and Risley (1968). This article, a landmark in the early development of the field, described the application of behavior principles and procedures with a wide variety of subjects, conditions, and environments. In addition, the authors discussed the techniques considered up-to-date at the time, such as training in the natural setting, using naturally occurring reinforcers, and employing a variety of these procedures we have now come to recognize as crucial for the facilitation of generalization.

The present volume serves as a transition from the accomplishments of the past (summarized in Kazdin's book) to the most current application of behavioral approaches. As a self-appointed judge of the major advances reported in the present volume during the past decade, it appears to me that the following developments represent significant new territory for both researchers and practitioners:

1. *Behavioral diagnostics*. The process of systematically arranging antecedent and consequent events while rewarding behavior offers practitioners the most accurate means of determining the causes of behavior and defining its relationship to environmental factors. Behavioral diagnostics goes beyond the assumption that the environment includes all of the conditions and events that are important for intervention. This approach recognizes that—particularly with individuals who have severe behavior disorders—certain physiological variables can have a real influence on behavior. These variables include the experience of physical discomfort, the inability to effectively signal a condition of deprivation, the symptoms of allergies, and the side effects of medication.

2. *Positive programming*. In positive programming, the teacher implements an instructional program that provides the student with the knowledge and the competence to interact with friends and peers in school and the wider community. This approach emphasizes the differential reinforcement of positive behaviors that facilitate social integration. Positive pro gramming procedures will become increasingly important as behaviorists strive to avoid the use of aversive stimuli in behavior management.

3. *Self-management*. Strategies of self-management encourage the involvement of the individual in the monitoring and control of his or her own behavior, which results in increased functional independence and stability. While this has always been the ultimate goal of all effective teaching and behavior intervention, we can now proceed more directly to arrange contingencies that build and strengthen the ability to manage and monitor the individual's own behavior.

4. *Parent training*. Current methods of parent training and direct involvement are indications of tremendous progress from the primitive, dynamic model presented by Bettelheim in *Love is Not Enough* (1950). Bettelheim strongly believed in removing and isolating parents from the treatment of their children. Modern behavior management, on the other hand, recognizes that parents are a critical part of the intervention process. The family provides the nexus for learning, with parents as the models for the behavior of the child. The family whose members have received training in applying behavior management has a distinct advantage over one that

employs random strategies or methods passed down from previous generations of parenting.

Even though I have identified these issues and areas of distinct progress for the 1980s and beyond, I do not mean to discount the valuable information and commentary on other topics made by the contributors to this volume. Indeed, the entire monograph provides an excellent and necessary source of information for all of us who are engaged in the teaching and management of children and youth who have severe behavior disorders.

In addition to these developments, there are several other issues that will be important for future directions in the field of behavior management. PL 99-457 (Education of the Handicapped Amendments of 1986) emphasizes the least restrictive environment for the early placement and education of all children and youth with handicaps. This means that children with serious behavior disorders must receive their schooling in regular classrooms along with other children, a necessary first step toward their ultimate inclusion in society. Teachers of these children should therefore work to facilitate peer interactions in the classroom. One of the most effective ways to do this is to set up positive programming that enlists normally developing children as both tutors and behavior models for children with severe behavior disorders. Classroom programs would emphasize peer academic tutoring and the appropriate social behavior for peer interactions. This new trend has proven to be beneficial for integrating children with behavior disorders into regular programs. It offers a successful direction for promoting peer involvement as well as the advantages of combining academic and social learning opportunities in the classroom.

Also important for the future is the systematic application of behavior analysis in the classroom, the results of which will lead to advances in the effectiveness of instruction. The collection of classroom data will continue to serve as the essential prerequisite for making instructional decisions. Through the data-based decision-making process, the research-oriented teacher can increase the rate at which students acquire new skills and determine when adequate levels of skill performance are achieved. Educators can also use this process to promote the generalization of skills, to ensure that skills learned in the training setting manifest themselves in other environments. The field of behavior modification has provided the framework for analyzing and measuring student performance in order to facilitate skill learning and generalization, and these procedures will continue to be important for making data-based instructional decisions. Behavior analysis applied in the classroom can help us achieve a research program that will contribute to more effective intervention and instruction.

Along with the refinement of instructional technology and its application, another major achievement during the last 20 years has been changes in the practices of educators, therapists, counselors, and school psychologists, all of whom have increased their levels of sophistication in applying behavioral principles in the exercise of their skills. The field of cognitive behavioral modification has provided the kind of compromise that many practitioners find comfortable as they proceed to change the behaviors of their students.

Cognitive behavioral strategies will continue to offer advantages in providing ways to build programs that apply self-mediation, monitoring, and self-management. If we assume a hierarchy of learning stages, during the first stages the individual acquires appropriate social behavior and demonstrates that behavior in a variety of environments; during the final application stage, the individual, when presented with a problem, quickly identifies the critical stimuli and takes appropriate steps to solve that problem. The final stage of effectively adapting to a variety of environments involves the highest level of self-mediation, monitoring, and management.

REFERENCES

Baer, D., Wolf, M., & Risley, T. (1968). Some current dimensions of applied behavior analysis. *Journal of Applied Behavior Analysis, 1,* 1, spring.

Bettelheim, B. (1950). *Love is not enough.* Glencoe, IL: Free Press.

Kazdin, A. E. (1978). *History of behavior modification.* Baltimore: University Park Press.

Introduction

Ennio Cipani
University of the Pacific

Behavior problems, in one form or another, concern almost all personnel in the developmental disabilities field. Discipline/behavior problems have commonly been cited as a major factor in staff turnover and "burnout," as well as in the failure to maintain clients in less restrictive educational and residential environments. Concerns regarding the management of severe behavioral problems can cause problems for even the best trained personnel.

Since the mid-1960s, applied behavior analysis research has focused on the management of behavior problems. The results of early investigations were encouraging, but generalizations were limited because these studies employed the case study approach to institutionalized subjects, with a limited number of settings and target behaviors. Additionally, treatment procedures focused primarily on reinforcement and punishment contingencies. Since that time, the research has expanded rapidly, involving the study of a variety of clinical populations in a variety of settings with varied target behaviors. The research has utilized extensive treatment packages and procedures in addition to redesigned contingencies. The progress that has occurred since the initial research has been substantial. However, certain areas related to both research and practice have not been adequately addressed. The effectiveness of this technology must be reviewed for personnel in developmental disabilities. This monograph serves as a source book for personnel in the field dealing with behavior problems.

The monograph covers a wide variety of behavioral approaches to the treatment of aberrant behavior. Developing technologies are presented and reviewed as well as updates on more researched programming efforts and procedures.

This volume is divided into three sections. The first section includes reviews and discussions of different approaches to the treatment of severe behavior problems. Within this first section, five different approaches are presented. Two treatment approaches that have been heavily researched over the past several decades—token economies and punishment—are presented. Techniques that have been heavily researched are reviewed and suggestions for practice and future research are delineated.

The token economy as a program for delivery contingencies has been a staple of behavioral practice, particularly in classrooms. As Williams, Williams, and McLaughlin point out in this chapter, there has been a great deal of research demonstrating its efficacy. Despite the empirical basis and advantages of using token economies to treat behavior problems, the usage of token economies is not as widespread as the empirical evidence regarding its efficacy would suggest. After reading this chapter, one may come to the conclusion that sometimes the "solution of the future" might be a better understanding and usage/application of an already existing technology.

Self-control strategies have been utilized more frequently with other populations, as Gardner and Cole point out in their chapter. The research on self-monitoring strategies with people with developmental disabilities is not extensive at this time. Therefore, their usage with people with developmental disabilities to treat behavior problems represents a behavioral technique that is not at the experimental stage of development, but does involve a new application of an already existing technology. It would seem that the application of this technology to people with developmental disabilities would require research to determine whether variables that affect treatment outcome in other populations would have similar effects in this field. While more research is warranted before such technology becomes a truly viable product for intervention, this chapter points to early results in the literature that are very promising.

Punishment techniques have also been utilized in everyday practice and heavily researched. The use of these techniques pervades life in all aspects. Yet, as O'Brien points out in this section, punishment is often misunderstood in terms of basic behavioral principles and as a result is often misapplied. So often, the clinical application of therapeutic punishment violates basic principles validated in laboratory research regarding its use and thereby compromises its effectiveness. This paper reviews basic principles of punishment validated in earlier laboratory research and then presents the research literature of a number of techniques. By providing personnel in the field with such information, it is hoped that a better understanding of the basic principles involved in punishment would occur and thereby render its use when clinically indicated more effective and decrease abusive practices. Again, solving future problems will rely in part on the applied field using already existing validated techniques in a more efficient fashion.

The last two chapters in this section represent newly emerging behavioral technologies for treating severe behavior problems. Positive programming can probably best be characterized as a package treatment approach to solving behavior problems based in large part on functional analysis of the problematic behavior. Increasingly, the behavior analyst of the 1980s and 1990s wants to know why a behavior is caused and, minimally, why it is maintained in level of occurrence. As LaVigna, Willis, and Donnellan present, many treatment strategies used in applied settings are reactive, while long-term solution requires a strategy that is proactive. Positive programming places great emphasis on developing functional appropriate alternative communicative behaviors, as well as generating ecological manipulations that alter the antecedent environment to change problematic behavior. The future thrust of research and clinical efforts would seem to be in the direction of nonaversive procedures; such empirical validation is needed if this emerging technology is to stand the behavioral analysis "litmus test."

Along the lines of the above chapter, Bailey and Pyles provide additional coverage on the use of behavioral diagnostic procedures to determine what the cause of the problem is. This diagnostic approach should be differentiated from traditional diagnostic approaches. A behavioral diagnostic approach would center on the analysis of environmental events that increase or decrease the likelihood of certain behaviors occurring.

In the second section, both chapters examine the research and practice in behavioral approaches to treating the respective problem behaviors. While the reinforcement and punishment procedures have been heavily utilized in treating aggressive and disruptive behavior, Danforth and Drabman point out that a behavioral approach at its optimum involves two types of analyses before treatment prescription: (a) a functional analysis of behavior and (b) an analysis of behavioral covariation. Similarly, Koegel and Koegel point out that nonaversive procedures, both antecedent and consequent strategies, are the "avant garde" of behavioral approaches of the 1990s for self-stimulatory behavior. Their chapter on community-referenced approaches to treatment highlights effective procedures that meet two standards of behavior analysis: the treatment strategy must be effective and it must be feasible for the setting(s) in which it will be utilized.

After reading the previous chapters, one might wonder why the field is not more adept at dealing with severe behavior problems. Certainly these chapters offer a substantial body of literature that provides empirical evidence that severe behavior problems can be brought under control and replaced by more socially appropriate behaviors. One does not have to look far for an answer: program implementation! Behavioral treatment approaches are designed by behavioral analysts; however, they are often implemented by staff or parents who may be relatively naive with respect to the technology. Therefore, a crucial, primary job of any behavioral program designer/consultant is to develop a behavioral repertoire in significant others and reinforce them for the utilization of such procedures. Hence, the need for the last two chapters.

The last two chapters of this monograph focus on the field's current understanding of developing skills in parents and personnel who work directly with children, adolescents, and adults with developmental disabilities. The importance of these two chapters cannot be overstressed because almost all treatment programs rely on people currently involved with the client to deliver intervention services. Given this fact, one must consider the extent to which a behavioral program designer can modify the existing repertoires of the current staff or parents.

As Egel and Powers point out, the idea of training parents in behavior modification to intervene in child problems in the home and community has been around for the past two decades. However, this is not to say that the field's approach to such a task has not evolved. As pointed out in this chapter, earlier clinical and research efforts centered around unidimensional approaches to solving a behavior problem in the home. Currently, behavioral strategies stressing a systems approach are favored, with the advocacy to begin empirical validation of such an approach. Behavioral approaches in general are becoming more involved in studying the ecological needs and ramifications of proposed interventions, and the field of parent training certainly seems to be in synchrony with such developments.

Training staff in behavioral techniques is a necessary, but not sufficient, condition for staff performance of behavioral techniques. As Reid, Parsons, and Green point out, getting staff to perform effectively requires more than just administrative memos. Rather, one must define performance responsibilities, monitor staff performance, teach new skills, and set up a performance feedback/consequence system. These authors are well suited to write a chapter on the state of the art in behavioral organizational management because they confront the problems involved in training staff in behavioral procedures and maintaining such skills over time at a large institution in North Carolina.

A monograph such as this one provides the reader with a resource on current treatment approaches to problematic behaviors. The capability of the technology has been demonstrated over the past several decades, with both procedures and problem assessments becoming more precise and conceptually refined. The field has come a long way from its early work with people with developmental disabilities. The strides in the development of future technological innovations will come in two areas: increased refinements of assessment and treatment techniques that match treatments to the function of the target problem, and increased attention to the development and maintenance of skills in personnel who work directly with the children in their natural environments (parents, peers, teachers, care providers, siblings, etc.).

The contributors to this volume are all experts in behavior analysis and enthusiastic advocates of the theoretical formulations and technologies they review in this text. The author, fully cognizant of the controversies surrounding the treatment of severe behavior disorders, has deliberately sought out diverse points of view for purposes of exposure, scholarship and debate in the open forum presented by the AAMR Monograph Series.

As of the date of this publication, the AAMR has adopted a position statement on aversive treatment, which states as follows:

Some persons who have mental retardation or developmental disabilities continue to be subjected to inhuman forms of aversive therapy techniques as a means of behavior modification. The American Association on Mental Retardation (AAMR) condemns such practices and urges their immediate elimination. The aversive practices to be eliminated include some or all of the following characteristics:

1. obvious signs of physical pain experienced by the individual;
2. potential or actual physical side-effects, including tissue damage, physical illness, severe stress, and/or death; and
3. dehumanization of the individual, through means such as social degradation, social isolation, verbal abuse, techniques inappropriate for the individual's age, and treatment out of proportion to the target behavior, because the procedures are normally unacceptable for nonhandicapped individuals.

The AAMR urges continuing research into humane methods of behavior management and support of existing programs and environments that successfully habilitate individuals with complex behaviors. (Adopted by the AAMR Board of Directors, December, 1986.)

Treatment Approaches

The Use of Token Economies With Individuals Who Have Developmental Disabilities

Betty Fry Williams,
Randy Lee Williams,
and Thomas F. McLaughlin

Gonzaga University
Department of Education

A considerable body of research concerning the effectiveness of token economies exists (Axelrod, 1971; Ayllon & Azrin, 1968b; Kazdin, 1977, 1982; Kazdin & Bootzin, 1972; McLaughlin & Williams, 1988; O'Leary & Drabman, 1971). The present review examined the educational and psychological research, specifically for applications of token economies with people with mental retardation, autism, and other developmental disabilities. This review considered (a) strategies for implementing token systems, (b) advantages of token economies, (c) instances of token implementation with people with developmental disabilities, and (d) reasons for the lack of use of token economies.

IMPLEMENTATION STRATEGIES

Theoretical Framework

A token is a generalized conditioned reinforcer that is distinguished by its physical properties (Skinner, 1953). Tokens are objects or symbols that in and of themselves probably have little or no reinforcing value (Axelrod, 1971), symbols or items that can be exchanged for primary or other conditioned reinforcers. The pairing of tokens and positive reinforcers during the exchange produces a conditioning effect (Skinner, 1953). The token itself takes on reinforcing value.

A token program involves the designation of the token, the selection of probable reinforcers (backups) for which the token may be exchanged, and the rules and rates by which tokens may be earned, lost, or spent. The most important example of a token economy in our society is the monetary system (O'Leary & Drabman, 1971). A great deal of behavior is maintained by the weekly or monthly paycheck; the paycheck itself is exchanged for goods and services of value to the individual. Occasionally, inappropriate behavior may be consequated by the loss of money, as when one is fined for a traffic violation. It is important to the success of the monetary system that money be obtained and exchanged only in authorized ways.

Types of Tokens

The tangible item or symbol that has been used as a token has varied considerably. Poker chips have been widely chosen and were even used in the earliest studies with chimps in 1936 and 1937 (O'Leary & Drabman, 1971). Poker chips have several practical advantages (McLaughlin & Williams, 1988). They stack easily, are highly visible, and the colors can be used to reflect different values. Other tokens have included heart-shaped paper punches (Aitchison & Green, 1974), red check marks (Bath & Smith, 1974), points (Broden, Hall, Dunlap, & Clark, 1970; McLaughlin, 1981; McLaughlin & Malaby, 1972a, 1975, 1976), stars (Buckingham, McLaughlin, & Hunsaker, 1978), aluminum discs (Burchard, 1967; Burchard & Barrera, 1972), clicks on a hand counter (Chaing, Iwata, & Dorsey, 1979), plastic interlocking links (Iwata & Bailey, 1974), currency (Logan, 1970; Payne, Polloway, Kauffman, & Scranton, 1975), and lottery tickets (Muir & Milan, 1982).

There are advantages to using tangible tokens (Ayllon & Azrin, 1968b). These include the direct relationship of the number of tokens to the amount of reward, the portability of tokens to other settings, and the ability to use tokens to operate automatic vending machines. Tangible tokens also provide a visible record of improvement (Kazdin & Bootzin, 1972). When selecting tangible tokens one should keep in mind the durability of the item, the ease with which the token can be standardized, and the ease with which the token can be protected from unauthorized duplication (Ayllon & Azrin, 1968b).

To be easily used, tokens should have the following properties: they should be easy to dispense and draw little attention away from the task at hand; they should have understandable value, and if possible, relate to real currency; they should be easy to transport to an exchange area and require little bookkeeping; they should be identifiable as the property of a specific individual; and they should be dispensable frequently enough to shape behavior (O'Leary & Drabman, 1971).

Backup Reinforcers

The backup reinforcers used in token programs have also varied widely. Most commonly used were candy, small toys, and trinkets (O'Leary & Drabman, 1971). Usually these tokens have been exchanged at a small store or actual commissary. Tokens have also been exchanged for free play time (Baer, Rowbury, & Baer, 1973), social outings (Bijou, Birnbrauer, Kidder, & Tague, 1966), privileges such as early lunch, restroom time, and moving desks (Broden et al., 1970), household merchandise and restaurant coupons (Muir & Milan, 1982), and watching television (Nordquist & Wahler, 1973). In studies in institutional facilities, the backups included access to privacy, religious services, movies, concerts, clothing, beauty items, smoking items, recreational activity, and so on (Atthowe & Krasner, 1968; Ayllon & Azrin, 1965; Burchard, 1967; Girardeau & Spradlin, 1964). In some classroom studies, backup items were free classroom activities easily available to any teacher, such as sharpening pencils, seeing animals, taking out balls, participating in sports, writing on the board, being on a committee, playing games, listening to records, coming into the room early, seeing the teacher's gradebook, and working on special jobs or projects (McLaughlin & Malaby, 1972a, b).

Tokens acquire their generalized conditioned reinforcing strength through pairing with a variety of backups during exchange periods. With individuals with developmental disabilities it has been critical that the initial pairings be with powerful reinforcers, occur frequently, and immediately follow the period of time during which the individual earned the tokens (McLaughlin & Williams, 1988). O'Leary and Drabman (1971) suggested, for example, that with children with mental retardation one may first have to establish the value of a token by repeatedly exchanging the token for a known reinforcer such as candy. Kazdin and Bootzin (1972) found that this was typically accomplished by giving out a few tokens immediately prior to the exchange time. Birnbrauer and Lawler (1964) established their token system with pupils with severe retardation by first reinforcing behavior with M&Ms, then consequating behaviors with tokens that could be immediately traded for M&Ms. The researchers then gradually increased the number of tokens required for each M&Ms exchange.

In order to increase the likelihood that the backup would have reinforcing value, some researchers have allowed individuals to choose the backup item prior to actually earning the tokens (Kazdin & Geesey, 1980; McGee, Krantz, & McClannahan, 1985; Neef, Walters, & Egel, 1984). Another way to determine whether a backup is actually a reinforcer is simply to observe what the individual spends free time doing (Premack, 1965) and designate this activity as a contingently earned backup. Ayllon and Azrin (1968a) also demonstrated a way to increase the effectiveness of backups through a technique called *reinforcer sampling*. They found that a particular backup activity was chosen more often when residents were exposed briefly to the stimuli associated with the backup activity. For example, residents were assembled outside the ward building and then asked if they would like to spend tokens on a walk outdoors. Reinforcer sampling helped to ensure that a variety of backups were paired with the tokens.

ADVANTAGES OF TOKEN
ECONOMIES

Token economies have been shown to be effective in increasing and maintaining behavior across a variety of populations and settings, including normal children in the regular classroom, handicapped students in special education classrooms, residents in psychiatric institutions, and legal offenders in detention (Kazdin, 1977). Many advantages of token economies have been cited. Kazdin (1977) and Kazdin and Bootzin (1972) have enumerated these advantages:

1. Tokens have been proven to be potent reinforcers; they have maintained behavior at higher levels than did praise, approval, and feedback alone.
2. Tokens have bridged the gap between the emission of a target behavior and its backup reinforcer. Tokens have mediated the delay between response and reinforcer and have allowed behavior to be maintained over a longer period of time.
3. Because tokens could be exchanged for a variety of backups, their reinforcing effect was less subject to deprivation and satiation states.
4. Tokens could be easily administered and given less disruptively than reinforcers that required consumption or activity.
5. Tokens permitted the administration of a standardized reward to a variety of individuals who had different reinforcer preferences. For example, poker chips could be given to all students during a lesson but they could be traded later for any of the several backups.
6. Tokens allowed for the parceling out of reinforcers that would otherwise be given on an all or nothing basis.
7. Tokens were practical for carrying and counting and provided a tangible record of progress.

Other advantages of token economies have also been cited:

1. Tokens have been sufficiently powerful to contain disruptive behavior so that other aversive procedures such as timeout could be substantially reduced (Birnbrauer, Wolf, Kidder, & Tague, 1965; Burchard, 1967).
2. Tokens provided an unambiguous indication of approval independent of the attendant's or teacher's particular personality or mood at the time of delivery (Ayllon & Azrin, 1965; Birnbrauer & Lawler, 1964).
3. Token economies reduced the need to discover what would reinforce the individual's behavior at the time when the response occurred.

It was necessary only to deliver the tokens and allow the individual to express personal preferences at the time of token exchange (Ferster, 1961).

4. The effectiveness of token reinforcement has not been restricted by age, intelligence, diagnosis, or history of institutionalization (Ayllon & Azrin, 1965).

5. Tokens could be paired with social feedback such as praise, smiling, and teacher attention to make these events effective reinforcers as well (Axelrod, 1971; Hewett, Taylor, & Artuso, 1969; Locke, 1969).

6. When carefully administered, tokens could assist in the generalization of behaviors to other settings, teacher/trainers, and times (Fowler & Baer, 1981; Kazdin & Bootzin, 1972; Mayhew & Anderson, 1980; O'Leary & Drabman, 1971).

7. Token economies provided a unique opportunity to investigate the effects of various reinforcement values and schedules on humans. One study manipulated token values to determine the effects on behavior (Schroeder, 1972), and others manipulated schedules to increase transfer (Touchette & Howard, 1984) and to increase resistance to extinction (Kazdin & Polster, 1973).

These numerous advantages of token economies have made them very attractive for implementation with special populations such as those with developmental disabilities.

TOKEN IMPLEMENTATION

Token economies have been applied with people with developmental disabilities in four general skill categories. Tokens have been used to establish academic skills in classroom settings including the development of attending to task, accuracy in reading, writing, language, and arithmetic, and answering questions. Tokens have also been used in classrooms and residential settings to establish compliance with instructions and expected social conduct. Speech and language instruction has also been carried out using tokens. The last area, which also represented the earliest work with token economies, included the development of daily living skills, self-help skills, and social interaction.

Academic Skills

The most basic of academic skills, attention to task, has been successfully acquired and maintained through token contingencies. Broden et al. (1970) compared the effects of teacher attention to the effects of tokens contingent on the study behavior of junior high school special education students. They found that social reinforcement could maintain study behavior at about 57%, but the use of contingent points raised maintained study behavior to 83%. The points were exchangeable for early lunch, permission to be out of seats, to move desks, to get a drink of water, to earn snacks, and to complete approved activities such as knitting or putting together puzzles. They also noted that as study behavior increased, disruptive behavior decreased.

Hewett et al. (1969) evaluated the use of the "engineered classroom" with children with emotional disturbance. Students earned checkmarks for starting work and staying on task. Checkmarks were exchanged for tangibles on a weekly basis. The authors found that contingent social approval alone was not initially as effective for maintaining attention to task as when social approval was paired with tokens. Once the students had experienced the token system, the token economy could be removed and behavior maintained with social contingencies alone. The researchers concluded that the token economy actually was useful in establishing control of behavior with social reinforcement. Because the tokens increased attention to task, an added effect was the improvement of arithmetic achievement.

Shapiro and Klein (1980) explored the use of tokens in the development of self-management skills of children with mental retardation and emotional disturbance in a psychiatric hospital school. As the children completed preacademic skills such as color and shape matching, they were given tokens for on-task behavior in random intervals of 30, 60, and 90 seconds. A bell rang to indicate token delivery, at which time the teacher would ask, "Were you working when the bell rang?" Tokens were given for on-task behavior and students were provided feedback on the accuracy of their self-assessment. Teacher instructions and prompts were gradually eliminated as the children learned to take tokens on their own at the sound of the bell if they had been on task throughout the interval. The researchers found that on-task behavior was significantly increased, off-task behavior was reduced by 50%, task accuracy and performance also increased, and students were successful in self-managing their own token contingencies.

Knapczyk and Livingston (1973) used self-recording with students with mental retardation in a junior high special education room. Students were given tokens for answering questions about the reading assignment. They recorded their own data, received toy money for completing requirements, and exchanged the token money at the end of the week for educational activities. Accuracy on answers to reading questions was increased with the token economy and the management of the token system was easily transferred to a student teacher.

Bijou et al. (1966) used tokens to maintain performance by children with retardation in programmed instruction in reading, writing, and math. Their 3-year study demonstrated that tokens established increased responding in contrast to verbal forms of approval, which initially had no effect. When the token system was removed, some of the students maintained rates of responding even without the tokens and others continued to perform above baseline levels, though at a reduced rate. Bijou et al. (1966) concluded that the pairing of tokens and teacher comments had the positive effect of strengthening the reinforcer effectiveness of teacher praise. They recommended giving tokens (a) as soon as possible consequent to targeted behaviors, (b) for increasingly larger units of behavior, and (c) in close association with praise, for extending the conditioning effect. Similar results had been reported in the research by Birnbrauer et al. (1965).

Dalton, Rubino, and Hislop (1973) compared the use of tokens to praise in a summer school program for children with Down syndrome. Responses to DISTAR language and arithmetic programs (Englemann & Carnine, 1969; Englemann, Osborn, & Englemann, 1969) was followed by contingent praise on a continuous schedule for one group and with tokens on an intermittent schedule accompanied by praise on a continuous schedule in the second group. The token group showed greatly superior performance in math during the study and a year later at followup.

Dixon (1981) used token reinforcement with nonverbal adolescents with severe retardation in developing picture-matching skills. The tokens were exchanged for small edibles and liquids. Touchette and Howard (1984) were also successful in using tokens to teach students with severe retardation and multiple handicaps to visually discriminate both letters and words.

Compliance

Many students with developmental disabilities do not cooperate under usual classroom conditions. Birnbrauer and Lawler (1964) found that a token economy could help children with severe behavior problems function in a group setting. Initially, compliance with a verbal request or exhibiting appropriate classroom behavior was rewarded with M&Ms. Later tokens were contingently earned and could be traded for the candy. Using a token system, Birnbrauer and Lawler were able to teach a student with profound retardation to sit quietly for about 60 minutes at a table with six other children; to hang up, put on, and zip a coat upon request; and to respond to the verbal requests "sit down," "close the door," and "don't touch." By the end of the year this student was able to begin discriminating pictures and colors, rarely attacked another child, and was seldom self-destructive.

The inappropriate behavior of children with moderate retardation was reduced by delivery of tokens contingent on the nonoccurrence of the undesired behaviors (Poling, Miller, Nelson, & Ryan, 1978). Although verbal reprimands had been ineffective, the differential token reinforcement of other than the undesired behavior was effective in reducing hands near mouth, drooling, leaving seat, hitting others, and throwing objects.

Response cost—the removal of tokens for undesirable behavior—has also been found to be effective in reducing disruptive behavior. Iwata and Bailey (1974) compared the effects of both token reward and response cost on rule violation behavior with elementary school special education children. During one phase, tokens were earned as long as no rule violations had occurred. During the other phase, a set number of tokens was given at the beginning of the session and tokens were lost, one at a time, for rule violations. Tokens were traded on "Surprise Day," which occurred at random times, for inexpensive toys and candy. Iwata and Bailey found that both procedures were about equally effective in reducing rule violations and off-task behavior. They also found that the rate of completing math problems doubled, while accuracy maintained at about 80%. No negative side effects of response cost were noted.

Burchard (1967) established a token economy with antisocial adolescent boys with retardation. Contingent verbal praise failed to be effective with this group, but a token economy wherein tokens were earned for compliance in the school and workshop but lost for inappropriate behavior was effective for habilitation. Stealing, lying, cheating, fighting, property damage, and verbal assault were greatly reduced during the token condition. Burchard and Barrera (1972), using a token system with the same population, found that a "heavy" token loss (30 tokens response cost) was as effective at decreasing antisocial behaviors as was a "heavy" (30-minute) timeout.

Dougherty, Fowler, and Paine (1985), working with younger boys with mild retardation, found that a combination reward and cost token system was effective in controlling behavior on the playground. Points were awarded for positive interactions with peers, such as giving a compliment. Points were lost for negative interactions such as criticism, accusations, name calling, threats, rough bodily contact, and so on. Rule infraction was also consequated with token loss. Dougherty et al. also successfully taught peers to monitor the behavior of the target children and eventually taught the target children to self-monitor. A 3-month followup showed that some of the improved behavior still remained.

Baer et al. (1973) used tokens to develop instructional control over the classroom activities of three preschoolers who were disruptive and who demonstrated autistic mannerisms, language deficits, and negativism. The preschoolers earned tokens for compliance by choosing the work task suggested by the teacher. Zimmerman, Zimmerman, and Russell (1969) found that tokens could be delivered as a group contingency to control the following of instructions by a class of boys with mental retardation. They also found that praise paired with tokens was more effective than were tokens alone.

Fjellstedt and Sulzer-Azaroff (1973) found that latency for following directions could be decreased by token contingencies. The subject, a child with emotional disturbance, was removed from the regular class because he could not follow directions within a reasonable period of time. Tokens given for compliance within 5 minutes of a request reduced latency from its previous 30-minute average. The child learned to move promptly from classroom to classroom, to sit at his desk and prepare to work, to begin work, and to put items away promptly when requested. Russo and Koegel (1977) were able to integrate an autistic child into a normal public school classroom by awarding tokens for compliance behaviors and removing tokens for self-stimulation. The regular classroom teacher was able to manage and then fade the use of tokens, so that control was maintained by social praise alone.

Chaing et al. (1979) were successful in eliminating the disruptive bus behavior of a boy with mental retardation. The bus driver administered tokens by clicking a hand counter if the child behaved appropriately over a predetermined distance of the bus ride. Once the child arrived at home or school, the parent or teacher would exchange the tokens earned for backups. Disruptive behavior on the bus was substantially reduced.

Language Skills

Children with developmental disabilities are frequently deficient in language skills. Consequently, a number of the studies using tokens with this population focused on the acquisition of either receptive and/or expressive language. McGee, Krantz, Mason, and McClannahan (1983) used a token economy to increase the receptive labeling of two adolescents with autism who had a long history of institutionalization. The girl and boy in the study learned to identify items they used in packing their school lunches. Tokens were later exchanged for food and drink. Buckingham et al. (1978) implemented a token system to increase the expressive language of an 11-year old child who was autistic. Using a changing criterion design, tokens were given for a complete sentence response to a question and later for a two-sentence response.

Neef et al. (1984) were able to establish yes/no responses in four preschoolers with developmental disabilities by using the token exchange time for embedded instruction. The children would choose the backup item they wished to earn prior to obtaining their tokens. Once the appropriate number of tokens had been earned and the child wished to exchange them for the preselected item, the teacher would use this opportunity to practice yes/no responses by asking questions like, "Is this what you wanted to buy?" and rewarding accurate yes or no responses. McGee et al. (1985) also used tokens with children with autism to establish expressive use of prepositions. The children were required to describe the locations of preferred edibles and toys for which they would later exchange their tokens.

Jackson and Wallace (1974) used a token economy to increase the loudness with which a teenaged girl with retardation spoke. A voice-operated relay was used that could only be activated by sufficient volume. Later, tokens were given contingent on polysyllabic words and then multiple words of sufficient volume. They found that the louder speech generalized to the classroom, although not to oral reading.

Baer and Guess (1971, 1973) successfully established the receptive use of particular morphemes with severely retarded adolescents. In their 1971 study, they used token rewards to establish the accurate identification of "-er" and "-est" endings for pictures showing, for example, *bigger* and *biggest* or *longer* and *longest*, and so forth. In the 1973 study, children with retardation were taught to convert verbs to nouns by adding the "-er" morpheme; for example, *run* became *runner*. The children earned poker chips that were traded at the end of each session for sweets and toys. The tokens demonstrated enough reinforcing strength to establish rather complex receptive and expressive skills.

Two language studies examined parents as treatment providers. Nordquist and Wahler (1973) trained the parents of a boy with multiple handicaps to reward verbal imitation with tokens. The tokens were then exchanged for brief units of television viewing. Muir and Milan (1982) actually applied the token system to the parents in their study. The mothers of three children with developmental disabilities earned lottery tickets and won prizes for the language progress made by their children. The children were to respond receptively to tasks, to imitate, and to label. For sufficient child progress, mothers were given lottery tickets from which there were drawings for household merchandise and restaurant meals. The lottery system was so successful that the improvement in the children's progress was clinically significant over progress under typical language therapy.

Daily Living Skills

Of paramount importance to individuals with developmental disabilities, particularly adults, is the acquisition of self-care and daily living skills. Girardeau and Spradlin (1964) awarded tokens to institutionalized adults with retardation for housework, self-care such as hair setting, group play, caring for animals, being on time, etc. Residents were so eager to earn tokens that the researchers were hard pressed to think of enough target behaviors. Winkler (1970) tested the impact of a token economy on chronic patients in a psychiatric ward. More than half of the women on the ward were termed "mental defectives." Winkler improved ward behaviors by rewarding attendance at an exercise program, completion of exercises, getting up, dressing, and making beds. Tokens were lost contingent on violence or loud noise such as screaming and tantrums. He found that when tokens were given noncontingently or when token fines were not given for inappropriate behaviors, patients' behaviors deteriorated. Bath and Smith (1974) found that a token economy on a ward for women with retardation improved social and life skills such as escorting others, teaching others to write, telling time, giving change, and so on. Martin, Pallotta-Cornick, Johnstone, and Goyos (1980) reported on the use of picture prompts in a sheltered workshop to increase production for institutionalized adults with retardation. These residents earned tokens for their work and exchanged them at the end of each day.

Various self-help skills have been established with token systems. Horner and Keilitz (1975) task analyzed toothbrushing and successfully taught the skill to adolescents with retardation residing at a state hospital. Tokens for toothbrushing were exchanged for sugarless gum. Thompson, Braam, and Fuqua (1982) developed a complex chain of laundering skills for retarded men. They used color charts and shape cues to prompt appropriate sorting, washing, and drying of clothes. Tokens were initially given on a continuous schedule, then on a gradually thinned variable ratio schedule, and finally faded out entirely. Richman, Reiss, Bauman, and Bailey (1984) used checkmarks on a token card to teach menstrual care to women with mild retardation. The women engaged in a training package and were taught to discriminate appropriate instances for changing soiled underwear and sanitary napkins.

DISCUSSION

Despite the demonstrated effectiveness of token economies with people with developmental disabilities, there has been a striking lack of use of token programs with this population. Bailey, Shook, Iwata, Reid, and Repp (1986) compiled articles on behavior analysis published in the area of developmental disabilities in the *Journal of Applied Behavior Analysis* from 1968 to 1985. Of the 62 articles they selected, only four indicated the use of token systems. Most of the studies reprinted used contingent praise and/or contingent edibles as reinforcers. A few studies indicated that objects or activities were used to try to reinforce behaviors, but no token mediation was reported. Although the advantages of token economies have been clearly shown, several factors seem to have inhibited their use.

One concern regarding token economies has been the cost such proce-dures might entail. Actually, token systems have been quite economical. Studies reporting cost have indicated that literally thousands of immediate rewards were given away at costs of under $10.00 per individual per year (Birnbrauer & Lawler, 1964; Girardeau & Spradlin, 1964). Other studies have used only cost-free backups (McLaughlin & Malaby, 1972a, b).

A second criticism of token programs has been that once tokens have been used, children would expect to receive tangibles for any work that they did (O'Leary & Drabman, 1971). This problem might be minimized by emphasizing the use of reinforcers intrinsic to the learning environment, such as recess, privileges, and social interaction.

The overjustification hypothesis (Lepper & Greene, 1978) stated that an individual reinforced with tangibles for an activity would come to attri-bute engaging in the activity to the extrinsic reward. Therefore, if a tangible was no longer given, the activity would cease (Fisher, 1979; Kazdin, 1977). Several studies demonstrated that the sudden cessation of tokens certainly reduced activity in most cases, but not all subjects ceased responding (Birnbrauer et al. 1965; Hewett et al. 1969). Other researchers have re-sponded that tokens could be gradually withdrawn without serious loss of activity if the withdrawal were carefully planned (Shapiro & Klein, 1980; Thompson, Braam, & Fuqua, 1982).

Some studies with people with developmental disabilities have revealed that a few individuals were unresponsive to token economies (Kazdin & Bootzin, 1972). These included some individuals with mental retardation and autism. However, in all of the studies reviewed, most of the subjects learned a variety of behaviors as a result of token systems. It would seem more feasible to individualize programs for the few individuals not affected by the token system than to forfeit token use for the majority.

The legal system has probably influenced the rate of adoption of token economies (Berwick & Morris, 1974, Kazdin, 1982). Court decisions, which have determined that students and residents in treatment had constitutional rights to noncontingent access to many objects and activities, have under-mined the backup systems of some token economies (Martin, 1975). Grounds passes, privacy, food, etc., which were once earned as backups, now must be provided without behavioral stipulations. This should not put an end to token economies, although it does mean that teachers and therapists must be more careful and creative in choosing and naming incen-tives that are reinforcing.

The last objection against token economies seems in many ways to be the best argument for its use. That has been the issue of generalization (Stokes & Baer, 1977). Generalization could be programmed into the token system in several ways. Kazdin and Bootzin (1972) and O'Leary and Drab-man (1971) have noted that: (a) the behaviors to be reinforced should be those that would later be naturally maintained; (b) individuals in token programs should be instructed in self-assessment and self-management of their rewards; (c) parents, other relatives and staff should also consequate with tokens; (d) tokens should be used across various settings and situations; (e) tokens should always be paired with social approval; (f) tokens should be given with increasing delays between token earning and token spending; and (g) tokens and backups should be given intermittently and gradually withdrawn.

The effective use of token economies has been extended greatly in recent years in terms of populations, settings, and behaviors in which they have been applied (Kazdin, 1982). Token economies have been demonstrated to be very effective with individuals with developmental disabilities across many behaviors. However, the use of tokens with people who have developmental disabilities still appears in the literature infrequently, compared with the use of primary reinforcers. The prospects that token systems offer for powerful motivation, generalization, and delay of gratification justify much greater implementation and on a wider basis.

REFERENCES

Aitchison, R. R., & Green, D. R. (1974). A token reinforcement system for the large wards of institutionalized adolescents. *Behavior Research and Therapy, 12*, 181–190.

Atthowe, J. M., & Krasner, L. (1968). Preliminary report on the application of contingent reinforcement procedures (token economy) on a "chronic" psychiatric ward. *Journal of Abnormal Psychology, 73*, 37–43.

Axelrod, S. (1971). Token reinforcement programs in special classes. *Exceptional Children, 37*, 371–379.

Ayllon, T., & Azrin, N. H. (1965). The measurement and reinforcement of behavior of psychotics. *Journal of the Experimental Analysis of Behavior, 8*, 357–383.

Ayllon, T., & Azrin, N. H. (1968a). Reinforcer sampling: a technique for increasing the behavior of mental patients. *Journal of Applied Behavior Analysis, 1*, 13–20.

Ayllon, T., & Azrin, N. H. (1968b). *The token economy: A motivational system for therapy and rehabilitation.* New York: Appleton-Century-Crofts.

Baer, D. M., & Guess, D. (1971). Receptive training of adjectival inflections in mental retardates. *Journal of Applied Behavior Analysis, 4*, 129–139.

Baer, D. M., & Guess, D. (1973). Teaching productive noun suffixes to severely retarded children. *American Journal of Mental Deficiency, 77*, 498–505.

Baer, A. M., Rowbury, T., & Baer, D. M. (1973). The development of instructional control over classroom activities of deviant preschool children. *Journal of Applied Behavior Analysis, 6*, 289–298.

Bailey, J. S., Shook, G. L., Iwata, B. A., Reid, D. H., Repp, A. C. (Eds). (1986). *Behavior analysis in developmental disabilities 1968–1985 from the Journal of Applied Behavior Analysis.* Reprint Series, Volume 1.

Bath, K. E., & Smith, S. A. (1974). An effective token economy program for mentally retarded adults. *Mental Retardation, 12*, 41–44.

Berwick, P. T., & Morris, L. A. (1974). Token economies: Are they doomed? *Professional Psychology, 5*, 434–439.

Bijou, S. W., Birnbrauer, J. S., Kidder, J. D., & Tague, C. E. (1966). Programmed instruction as an approach to the teaching of reading, writing, and arithmetic to retarded children. *Psychological Record, 16*, 505–522.

Birnbrauer, J. S., & Lawler, J. (1964). Token reinforcement for learning. *Mental Retardation, 2*, 275–279.

Birnbrauer, J. S., & Wolf, M. M., Kidder, J., & Tague, C. E. (1965). Classroom behavior of retarded pupils with token reinforcement. *Journal of Experimental Child Psychology, 2*, 219–235.

Broden, M., Hall, R. V., Dunlap, A., & Clark, R. (1970). Effects of teacher attention and a token reinforcement system in a junior high school special education class. *Exceptional Children, 36*, 341–349.

Buckingham, H., McLaughlin, T. F., & Hunsaker, D. (1978). Increasing oral responses in a special education student with a token program. *Education and Treatment of Children, 1*, 19–24.

Burchard, J. D. (1967). Systematic socialization: A programmed environment for the habilitation of antisocial retardates. *Psychological Record, 17*, 461–467.

Burchard, J. D., & Barrera, F. (1972). An analysis of timeout and response cost in a programmed environment. *Journal of Applied Behavior Analysis, 5*, 271–282.

Chaing, S. J., Iwata, B. A., & Dorsey, M. F. (1979). Elimination of disruptive bus riding behavior via token reinforcement on a "distance-based" schedule. *Education and Treatment of Children, 2*, 101–109.

Dalton, A. J., Rubino, C. A., & Hislop, M. W. (1973). Some effects of token rewards on school achievement of children with Down's Syndrome. *Journal of Applied Behavior Analysis, 6*, 251–259.

Dixon, L. S. (1981). A functional analysis of photo-object matching skills of severely retarded adolescents. *Journal of Applied Behavior Analysis, 14*, 465–478.

Dougherty, S. B., Fowler, S. A., & Paine, S. C. (1985). The use of peer monitors to reduce negative interaction during recess. *Journal of Applied Behavior Analysis, 18*, 141–153.

Englemann, S., & Carnine, D. (1969). *DISTAR arithmetic 1: An instructional system*. Chicago: Science Research Associates.

Englemann, S., Osborn, J., & Englemann, T. (1969). *DISTAR language: An instructional system*. Chicago: Science Research Associates.

Ferster, C. B. (1961). Positive reinforcement and behavioral deficits of autistic children. *Child Development, 32*, 437–456.

Fisher, E. B. (1979). Overjustification effects in token economies. *Journal of Applied Behavior Analysis, 12*, 407–415.

Fjellstedt, N., & Sulzer-Azaroff, B. (1973). Reducing the latency of a child's responding to instructions by means of a token system. *Journal of Applied Behavior Analysis, 6*, 125–130.

Fowler, S. A., & Baer, D. M. (1981). "Do I have to be good all day?" The timing of delayed reinforcement as a factor in generalization. *Journal of Applied Behavior Analysis, 14*, 13–24.

Girardeau, F. L., & Spradlin, J. E. (1964). Token rewards in a cottage program. *Mental Retardation, 2*, 341–351.

Hewett, F., Taylor, F., & Artuso, A. (1969). The Santa Monica project: Evaluation of an engineered classroom design with emotionally disturbed children. *Exceptional Children, 35*, 523–529.

Horner, R. D., & Keilitz, I. (1975). Training mentally retarded adolescents to brush their teeth. *Journal of Applied Behavior Analysis, 8*, 301–309.

Iwata, B. A., & Bailey, J. S. (1974). Reward versus cost token systems: An analysis of the effects on students and teacher. *Journal of Applied Behavior Analysis, 7*, 567–576.

Jackson, D. A., & Wallace, F. R. (1974). The modification and generalization of voice loudness in a fifteen-year-old retarded girl. *Journal of Applied Behavior Analysis, 7*, 461–471.

Kazdin, A. E. (1977). *The token economy: A review and evaluation*. New York: Plenum Press.

Kazdin, A. E. (1982). The token economy: A decade later. *Journal of Applied Behavior Analysis, 15*, 431–446.

Kazdin, A. E., & Bootzin, R. R. (1972). The token economy: An evaluative review. *Journal of Applied Behavior Analysis, 5*, 343–372.

Kazdin, A. E., & Geesey, S. (1980). Enhancing classroom attentiveness by preselection of back-up reinforcers in a token economy. *Behavior Modification, 4*, 98–114.

Kazdin, A. E., & Polster, R. (1973). Intermittent token reinforcement and response maintenance in extinction. *Behavior Therapy, 4*, 386–391.

Knapczyk, D. R., & Livingston, G. (1973). Self-recording and student supervision: Variables within a token economy structure. *Journal of Applied Behavior Analysis, 6,* 481–486.

Lepper, M. R., & Greene, D. (Eds.) (1978). *The hidden costs of reward: New perspectives on the psychology of human motivation.* New York: John Wiley & Sons.

Locke, B. (1969). Verbal conditioning with retarded subjects: Establishment or reinstatement of effective reinforcing consequences. *American Journal of Mental Deficiency, 73,* 621–626.

Logan, D. L. (1970). A "paper money" token system as a recording aid in institutional settings. *Journal of Applied Behavior Analysis, 3,* 183–184.

Martin, G., Pallotta-Cornick, A., Johnstone, G., & Goyos, C. (1980). A supervisory strategy to improve work performance for lower functioning retarded clients in a sheltered workshop. *Journal of Applied Behavior Analysis, 13,* 183–190.

Martin, R. (1975). *Legal challenges to behavior modification: Trends in schools, corrections and mental health.* Champaign, IL: Research Press.

Mayhew, G. L., & Anderson, J. (1980). Delayed and immediate reinforcement: Retarded adolescents in an educational setting. *Behavior Modification, 4,* 527–545.

McGee, G. G., Krantz, P. J., Mason, D., & McClannahan, L. E. (1983). A modified incidental-teaching procedure for autistic youth: Acquisition and generalization of receptive object labels. *Journal of Applied Behavior Analysis, 16,* 329–338.

McGee, G. G., Krantz, P. J., & McClannahan, L. E. (1985). The facilitative effects of incidental teaching on preposition use by autistic children. *Journal of Applied Behavior Analysis, 18,* 17–31.

McLaughlin, T. F. (1981). An analysis of token reinforcement: A control group comparison with special education youth employing measures of clinical significance. *Child Behavior Therapy, 3,* 43–51.

McLaughlin, T. F., & Malaby, J. (1972a). Intrinsic reinforcers in a classroom token economy. *Journal of Applied Behavior Analysis, 5,* 263–270.

McLaughlin, T. F., & Malaby, J. (1972b). Reducing and measuring inappropriate verbalizations in a token economy. *Journal of Applied Behavior Analysis, 5,* 329–333.

McLaughlin, T. F., & Malaby, J. E. (1975). The effects of token reinforcement contingencies on the completion and accuracy of assignments under fixed and variable token exchange schedules. *Canadian Journal of Behavioural Science, 7,* 411–417.

McLaughlin, T. F., & Malaby, J. E. (1976). An analysis of assignment completion across time during fixed, variable, and extended periods in a classroom token economy. *Contemporary Educational Psychology 1,* 346–355.

McLaughlin, T. F., & Williams, R. L. (1988). The token economy in the classroom. In J. C. Witt, S. N. Elliot, & F. M. Gresham (Eds.), *Handbook of behavior therapy in education.* New York: Plenum.

Muir, K. A., & Milan, M. A. (1982). Parent reinforcement for child achievement: The use of a lottery to maximize parent training effects. *Journal of Applied Behavior Analysis, 15,* 455–460.

Neef, N. A., Walters, J., & Egel, A. L. (1984). Establishing generative yes/no responses in developmentally disabled children. *Journal of Applied Behavior Analysis, 17,* 453–460.

Nordquist, V. M., & Wahler, R. G. (1973). Naturalistic treatment of an autistic child. *Journal of Applied Behavior Analysis, 6,* 79–87.

O'Leary, K. D., & Drabman, R. (1971). Token reinforcement programs in the classroom: A review. *Psychological Bulletin, 75,* 379–398.

Payne, J. S., Polloway, E. A., Kauffman, J. M., & Scranton, T. R. (1975). *Living in the classroom: A currency-based token economy.* New York: Human Sciences Press.

Poling, A., Miller, K., Nelson, N., & Ryan, C. (1978). Reduction of undesired classroom behavior by systematically reinforcing the absence of such behavior. *Education and Treatment of Children, 1,* 35–41.

Premack, D. (1965). Reinforcement theory. In D. Levine (Ed.), *Nebraska Symposia on Motivation.* Lincoln: University of Nebraska Press.

Richman, G. S., Reiss, M. L., Bauman, K. E., & Bailey, J. S. (1984). Teaching menstrual care to mentally retarded women: Acquisition, generalization, and maintenance. *Journal of Applied Behavior Analysis, 17,* 441–451.

Russo, D. C., & Koegel, R. L. (1977). A method for integrating an autistic child into a normal public-school classroom. *Journal of Applied Behavior Analysis, 10,* 579–590.

Schroeder, S. R. (1972). Parametric effects of reinforcement frequency, amount of reinforcement, and required response force on sheltered workshop behavior. *Journal of Applied Behavior Analysis, 5,* 431–441.

Shapiro, E. S., & Klein, R. D. (1980). Self-management of classroom behavior with retarded/disturbed children. *Behavior Modification, 4,* 83–97.

Skinner, B. F. (1953). *Science and human behavior.* Toronto: Macmillan.

Stokes, T. F., & Baer, D. M. (1977). An implicit technology of generalization. *Journal of Applied Behavioral Analysis, 10,* 349–367.

Thompson, T. J., Braam, S. J., & Fuqua, R. W. (1982). Training and generalization of laundry skills: A multiple probe evaluation with handicapped persons. *Journal of Applied Behavior Analysis, 15,* 177–182.

Touchette, P. E., & Howard, J. S. (1984). Errorless learning: Reinforcement contingencies and stimulus control transfer in delayed prompting. *Journal of Applied Behavior Analysis, 17,* 175–188.

Winkler, R. C. (1970). Management of chronic psychiatric patients by a token reinforcement system. *Journal of Applied Behavior Analysis, 3,* 47–55.

Zimmerman, E. H., Zimmerman, J., & Russell, C. D. (1969). Differential effects of token reinforcement on instruction following behavior in retarded students instructed as a group. *Journal of Applied Behavior Analysis, 2,* 101–112.

Self-Management Approaches

William I. Gardner
Waisman Center on Mental Retardation and Human Development
University of Wisconsin-Madison

Christine L. Cole
Lehigh University
Department of School Pyschology

INTRODUCTION

A review of the recent behavioral literature addressing treatment of aberrant behaviors in those with developmental disabilities reveals three distinct trends (Gardner & Cole, in press). The first is characterized by a decline in the number of published studies reporting the effects of various punishment procedures on aberrant behaviors. From the 1950s, when clinical researchers began investigating behavioral treatment of aberrant behaviors among this group, through the 1970s, a major focus has been on reducing or eliminating problem behaviors through presentation of contingent aversive consequences (Gardner, 1988). This focus reflected a ". . .consensus among researchers and clinicians that the elimination of behavior problems is an important first step in remediation" (Carr & Durand, 1985, p. 111). Comments by Repp and Brulle (1981) that "[T]he behavioral study of aggressive behavior has been to this date primarily a study of how to consequate behavior so that it will be rapidly reduced" (p. 206) and by Bornstein, Bach, and Anton (1982) that "[F]or the severely and profoundly retarded person, aversive procedures, and, to a lesser extent, time-out may be the treatment of choice" (p. 263) support this view. Even though the published literature of the 1980s continues to focus excessively on deceleration through aversive procedures (e.g., Foxx, McMorrow, Bittle, & Bechtel, 1986; Rolider & Van Houten, 1985), a distinct decline in punishment studies is evident.

Acknowledgment. Preparation of this paper was supported in part by Research Grant #G008300148 from the National Institute of Disability and Rehabilitation Research, Department of Education, Washington, DC 20202.

19

A second trend is represented by the increased emphasis on use of a behavioral diagnostic model as a basis for developing client-specific treatment procedures (Axelrod, 1987; Gardner & Cole, 1984, 1985, 1987). This diagnostic approach, in addition to evaluating influences residing in the external environment that may instigate, strengthen, or suppress behaviors, has focused attention on characteristics of the person that may contribute to the occurrence of inappropriate behaviors. As described by Gardner and Cole (1987), some of these personal characteristics (e.g., anger, chronic pain) may *by their presence* influence the probability that aberrant behaviors will occur. Other personal characteristics (e.g., social skill deficits, self-management deficits, motivational deficits) may *by their absence or low strength* increase the likelihood of aberrant behavior under provoking or stress conditions. The person may have limited or no alternative means of coping with sources of provocation. As a result, the person may engage in aberrant behavior in an attempt to remove or reduce the unwanted conditions (Carr & Newsom, 1985; Carr, Newsom, & Binkoff, 1980).

Studies that reflect this skill deficit perspective have focused on teaching alternative social/coping skills (e.g., Carr & Durand, 1985; Durand & Carr, 1987) and/or the skills to self-influence these in one way or another (e.g., Cole, Gardner, & Karan, 1985; Reese, Sherman, & Sheldon, 1984). These latter studies reflect the third trend in the behavior therapy literature: namely, an emphasis on teaching the person with mental retardation various skills of self-management as alternatives to the external management procedures that have dominated behavioral interventions. This trend is consistent with current legal guidelines for least restrictive treatment and reflects a basic ethical commitment to providing the most humane and normalizing treatment available. It also is consistent with the opposition to use of aversive procedures voiced by various professional organizations such as the American Association on Mental Retardation (Berkowitz, 1987) and The Association for Persons with Severe Handicaps (Guess, Helmstetter, Turnbull, & Knowlton, 1987). Finally, from both theoretical and pragmatic perspectives, this changing focus avoids some of the basic problems associated with excessive reliance on suppression of aberrant behaviors through use of aversive consequences and concurrently offers greater promise of producing behavior change of a more durable nature (Axelrod, 1987).

The value of teaching skills of self-management is further emphasized by recent requirements imposed on those with mental retardation to become increasingly independent and responsible for their own actions. With community residential, educational, and vocational placement, a reduction in external controls should occur in principle, if not in fact. In many instances, however, the person has not acquired the skills to assume responsibility for aspects of his or her own actions because of insufficient previous learning opportunities.

As is true in numerous areas of behavior therapy, the research and clinical application literature in self-management by those with mental retardation is significantly delayed relative to developments made with people without such cognitive and adaptive behavior difficulties (Gardner & Cole, 1988). This delay reflects the attitude that those with mental retardation are not capable of managing aspects of their own behavior. Additionally, until recently, the teaching of self-management has been inconsistent with the external control that is an integral component of institutional management. The reader is encouraged to consult Agran and Martin (1987) and Shapiro (1981, 1986) for discussion of additional factors that have impeded development in the application of self-management to those with mental retardation.

The majority of the self-management research has been concerned with teaching or improving various social (e.g., Matson & Andrasik, 1982), vocational (e.g., McNally, Kompik, & Sherman, 1984), self-help (e.g., Alberto, Sharpton, Briggs, & Stright, 1986), and academic (e.g., Shapiro, Browder, & D'Huyvetters, 1984) behaviors. In contrast, relatively minimal attention has been devoted to investigating the effects of self-management approaches on clinically significant aberrant behaviors displayed by persons with mental retardation. The research demonstrations involving self-management that are available to the practitioner usually are embedded in a multicomponent treatment package. As a result, clear demonstrations of the therapeutic contributions of specific individual self-management procedures have not been made. As will become evident, in a majority of the studies reported it can be said at best that the treatment programs (a) include self-management procedures and (b) are consistent with the philosophy of shifting behavioral control (responsibility) from the external environment to the person himself or herself.

The present chapter describes studies that support the potential efficacy of self-management procedures in reducing aberrant behaviors. These procedures, and the training programs used to teach these skills, are described in sufficient detail to provide the reader with a view of the specific modifications made to accommodate the cognitive and physical characteristics of the clients served. Although of importance, space restrictions do not permit discussion of the validity of the concept of self-management relative to its implied unique processes or motivation features. Independent of the question of why various self-management procedures influence a person's behavior (i.e., what may be the actual processes, mechanisms, or principles of behavioral influence), the procedures do have considerable user appeal and broader social validity. As noted, the procedures are highly consistent with a concept of independence as well as with the current focus on therapeutic interventions of a nonaversive nature. The appeal is especially attractive in treatment of the aberrant behaviors of those with mental retardation in view of the major historical emphasis on use of aversive procedures.

SELF-MANAGEMENT:
DEFINITION AND PROCEDURES

Self-management has reference to those behaviors engaged in by an individual that influence the likelihood of others of his or her own behaviors. Related to excessively occurring aberrant behaviors, self-management treatment refers to the person doing something (the controlling response) that would change the probability of occurrence of an inappropriate behavior (the controlled response) that currently has some strength of occurrence and is under some other controlling influences. These controlling self-management strategies include those that precede a target behavior (behavioral antecedents) as well as those that follow a target behavior (behavioral consequences). These procedures are listed in Table 1. The major focus of research on influencing aberrant behaviors of those with mental retardation has been on those procedures classified as behavioral consequences, specifically self-monitoring and self-consequation. While other procedures have been used, these typically are components of more comprehensive treatment packages.

TABLE 1

Self-Management Procedures

ANTECEDENTS		CONSEQUENCES	
Self	-instruction (cueing) -verbal -pictorial -prerecorded statements	Self	-monitoring -observation -discrimination -recording
Self	-selection of consequences	Self	-evaluation (assessment)

	-amount and type of reinforcers
	-amount and type of negative
	  consequences
		Self	-consequation (reinforcement;
			  punishment)

Self	-determined performance
	  criteria (standard setting)
		Self	-reinforcement
			-administration of self-selected
			  reinforcers
			-administration of reinforcers
			  determined by others

		Self	-punishment
			-administration of self-selected
			  negative consequences
			-administration of negative
			  consequences determined by
			  others

Self-Monitoring

Self-monitoring has been demonstrated to produce therapeutic reactive effects with individuals with diverse personal characteristics and behaviors (Gardner & Cole, 1988). The person, after determining the occurrence or nonoccurrence of a target behavior at a specific time or during a specific time period, makes a recording of this discrimination. This simple act of self-recording a self-discriminated behavior may result in a change in the occurrence of the behavior. Self-monitoring may be used as the only intervention procedure or may be combined with externally managed treatment approaches.

Self-Monitoring Used Alone

Self-Injurious Behaviors.   In one of the initial studies demonstrating reactivity of self-recording of an aberrant behavior by a person with mental retardation, Zegiob, Klukas, and Junginger (1978) trained an adolescent female with mild mental retardation to self-monitor nose and mouth picking (gouging). This behavior had caused severe swelling, bleeding, and redness of that facial area. Further, the picking interfered with the adolescent's speech and task performance. Previous attempts to eliminate the behavior through token programs and negative attention had been unsuccessful.

Training consisted of teaching the adolescent, through modeling and rehearsal, to identify the target behavior and to record the occurrence of each episode using a pencil and index card. Additionally, the inappropriateness of the target behavior was stressed and the client was prompted to name several negative aspects (e.g., it is unhealthy, it interferes with speech). Training occurred during an afternoon and evening session in the living environment in which the independent self-monitoring was to occur. Following training, the adolescent, on return to her living area in the afternoon, was provided a pencil and index card for self-recording. No further comments were made by staff regarding any aspects of the program. A reversal design was used to evaluate the effects of treatment. Following a second self-monitoring phase, the adolescent was praised hourly for "running her program." The program was faded over a 14-day period, with 3- and 6-month followup data obtained.

Following initiation of self-monitoring, an immediate reduction in the target was obtained (from 51.4 episodes per 15-minute intervals to 6.8 episodes). In the reversal phase, similar results were obtained (51.2 episodes to 9.6 episodes). With the addition of praise for running her program, the behavior was further reduced to 6.2 episodes. Additionally, a qualitative change was noted in that the nose and mouth gouging changed to touching her nose or mouth. During fading, occurrences decreased to 4.0 episodes. Three and 6-month followup revealed 2.5 and 2.0 episodes respectively.

Stereotyped Behavior.   Similar results were obtained with a 15-year-old female with moderate mental retardation who presented chronic stereotyped head shaking. Training and treatment, identical with that described previously, occurred during a 2½ hour period that included a language class, a free period, and a noon meal. Self-monitoring produced a therapeutic effect (62.5% of intervals observed spent in head shaking during initial baseline to 22.5% during self-monitoring). Following the addition of a procedure of daily charting of results and displaying these in the classroom, the behavior was further reduced to 2.5%, with some days completely free of the target behavior.

Self-Monitoring Combined with External Procedures

Reese et al. (1984) evaluated the effects of self-monitoring on the agitated disruptive behaviors of persons living in community group homes. The self-recording procedure was embedded in a multicomponent behavior therapy program. Its effects were evaluated by presenting and removing the self-management component, while maintaining all other program procedures.

In an initial evaluation of the program, a 22-year-old female functioning in the moderate range of mental retardation and demonstrating periodic incidents of agitated disruptive behaviors (e.g., yelling, cursing, kicking and banging and throwing objects, attacking staff) was taught to self-record the occurrence/nonoccurrence of the behaviors during designated time intervals. The client was provided a pocket timer and a recording sheet on which was listed the agitated-disruptive behaviors and a column of time intervals. Next to each time interval, marked off in hours, were two blanks marked either "Handled my temper" or "Lost my temper." After having been taught to set the pocket timer, the client then was instructed to mark her sheet in the appropriate blank when the timer sounded. The recording sheet was checked once per day against a similar record kept by a teaching counselor, and points were awarded both for recording correctly and for the nonoccurrence of agitated disruptive behaviors during an interval. Points were exchanged for a variety of reinforcers, including special activities such as trips to the movies or to eat.

As noted, the self-recording procedure represented an addition to ongoing token economy and related response cost procedures for agitated disruptive behaviors used in the client's group home. The client was also taught how to relax when she engaged in preagitated behaviors (rapid breathing and rapid, high-pitched speech). Additionally, she was taught a socially acceptable means of avoiding or escaping from situations that produced agitated disruptive behavior. When the client felt herself becoming upset, she was taught to maintain eye contact and, keeping a straight posture and facing the person upsetting her, to excuse herself, informing the person that she would like to talk later, and then engage in deep muscle relaxation experiences.

Use of the self-recording procedure coincided with a significant reduction in the frequency and duration of agitated disruptive behaviors. The writers, concluding that the self-recording procedure was an essential part of the treatment package, noted "the relatively immediate increase in agitated disruptive behavior on the two occasions when the self-recording procedure was eliminated makes it unlikely that unknown variables accounted for the change" (Reese et al., 1984, p. 97).

It is interesting to note that the client recorded correctly when she had not displayed agitated disruptive behavior, but never recorded correctly when she did exhibit agitated disruptive behaviors. Nonetheless, the self-recording procedure resulted in positive therapeutic effects. These results are consistent with the findings of other studies that accuracy of self-recording may not be critical to reactivity (Shapiro, 1986).

Reese et al. (1984) speculated, based on their observations that the client seemed to be using the self-recording procedure to recruit reinforcement, that the therapeutic effects observed derived from the social feedback provided by peers. This observation led these researchers to a similar study, in which a peer in the group home was responsible for reminding a second client, a 28-year-old female functioning in the upper moderate to lower mild range of mental retardation, to self-record the occurrence/nonoccurrence of her target disruptive agitated behavior every 2 hours. The peer was to praise the client and comment to others in the vicinity about how good the client had been. Additionally, points earned went toward a special outing for both the client and her peer assistant. Following demonstration of treatment effects, the self-recording intervals were increased to 4 hours and, during a maintenance phase, to 6 hours. Finally, at 6-month followup, results similar to those of the initial investigation were obtained. Self-recording seemed to exert a significant therapeutic effect (Reese et al., 1984). A third single-subject study demonstrated similar therapeutic effects of the program on agitated disruptive behaviors presented by a client in a workshop setting (Reese et al., 1984).

Self-Management Packages

In addition to studies in which self-monitoring is used as the self-management treatment component, other studies have evaluated the effects on aberrant behaviors of multiple self-management procedures combined into a package. These packages have been used both as treatment approaches to produce behavior change and as strategies to insure maintenance of behavior gains obtained initially from other externally managed therapy programs.

Self-Management: Treatment Strategies

Socially Undesirable Behaviors.   Rosine and Martin (1983) used a treatment program involving various self-management components to reduce the socially undesirable behaviors of young adults with mild to moderate levels of mental retardation. These adults, attending a sheltered workshop program, initially demonstrated chronic problems of tongue protrusion and tongue chewing. During individual training sessions, each client was initially provided evaluative statements regarding the inappropriateness of the target behavior, along with comments from the trainer that the client would learn not to engage in the behavior. Next, the client was trained to use a cumulative wrist counter. The self-monitoring procedure was modeled while the trainer performed the workshop task. To illustrate, the trainer modeled the target behavior (e.g., tongue protruding and chewing), verbalized a *self-instruction* (e.g., "Stop chewing your tongue!"), *self-recorded* (e.g., pressed the wrist counter), and then *self-praised* (e.g., "Good man!"). Following modeling, the client was prompted to rehearse the sequence previously observed. If the target behavior did not occur spontaneously, the trainer prompted its occurrence. Praise was provided by the trainer whenever the client engaged in the self-instruction, self-recording, and self-praise sequence. If these self-management behaviors did not occur, the trainer prompted the client to demonstrate these and then provided praise.

Following this training experience, the client was provided tokens and trained to exchange these for backup reinforcers. In subsequent sessions, the client was informed that a larger number of tokens would be earned by decreasing the target behavior. Following training sessions, the client next was trained to chart the scores obtained from the counter onto a frequency graph. It was emphasized again that a decreasing number of responses resulted in an increasing number of tokens. Training was transferred to the workshop and consisted of 1-hour sessions. During these, the trainer sat beside the client while the client was working. Praise was provided whenever the self-management sequence followed occurrence of the target. If self-management did not occur, the sequence was prompted by the trainer. Counter totals were charted, tokens provided based on performance, and tokens were exchanged for backup reinforcers.

Following this training, the client was given the responsibility to self-record target behaviors during half-day work sessions. Workshop staff were encouraged to praise any occurrence of the self-managed behaviors observed, to prompt it if observed not occurring following a target, and to remove the counter if observed being misused. Additionally, praise was provided for a session during which the target behavior did not occur. As during training, the client recorded and collected tokens at the end of each session. As a final step, the client was given responsibility for self-managing the target throughout the entire work day.

In a multiple baseline across subjects design, each of three clients demonstrated an immediate and significant reduction in the target behaviors, both while working in the workshop and during time in the kitchen or break room. Thus treatment effects generalized to locations in which no formal treatment occurred.

Stereotyped Behaviors.   Morrow and Presswood (1984) demonstrated the clinical usefulness of a self-management treatment package in reducing three stereotyped behaviors of a 15-year-old adolescent with multiple physical and psychological difficulties. This student, institutionalized for 3 years, had (a) a profound bilateral, sensorineural hearing loss, (b) a psychiatric diagnosis of schizophrenia and was described as frequently being out of contact with reality, and (c) a prorated Wechsler Intelligence Scale for Children-Revised IQ of 10.

Treatment occurred in the student's classroom, located in a state residential treatment center for mentally ill and behaviorally disordered children and youth. Although enrolled in a token economy program at the time of initiation of the self-management treatment program (tokens awarded every 30 minutes for being in the assigned area and completing academic assignments), staff reported no positive effects of the token system. Target behaviors consisted of (a) jaw and ear flapping with the palm of the hand, (b) hand contortions consisting of sudden closing and opening of the fist and inappropriate movement of the fist around the mouth, and (c) inappropriate shrieking noises when a response was not requested.

The adolescent was taught to self-monitor the occurrence of his behaviors during a predetermined time interval and to self-record on a grid the occurrence or nonoccurrence of the three target behaviors. During training, a timer was set to ring after a predetermined time interval. If the target behavior (e.g., jaw and ear flapping) had not occurred during the interval, an apparatus on his desk displayed a happy face and he was prompted to sign "I did not flap my ear or jaw" and record a plus (+) on a grid card located on his desk. The timer was reset and the adolescent was prompted to resume his assigned work, a match-to-sample vocabulary task. If a target behavior did occur before the timer rang, an unhappy face would be displayed and the adolescent would be prompted to sign "I did flap my ear or jaw" and record a minus (−) on the card. Training was continued until he was able to set the timer and correctly self-assess his target behaviors. No external reinforcement was provided. At the end of each daily session, the grid card was collected without feedback.

A multiple baseline across behaviors was used to assess the therapeutic effects of self-management treatment. Jaw and ear flapping reduced from a mean of 18.6 occurrences per 30 minutes during baseline to 0 in 8 days following treatment. The target did not occur during the remaining 33 days of data collection. Hand contortions showed a similar immediate reduction (mean of 12.4 per minute to 4 or fewer within 6 days and then to 0 episodes for the remaining days). Inappropriate noises also showed an immediate and significant reduction (83.4 episodes per 30 minutes during baseline to 17.2 following treatment initiation), although this behavior was not eliminated until an additional procedure of contingent exercise was introduced. To evaluate generalization of these treatment effects, probes were conducted for each of the three target behaviors in four school-related environments during the entire 5½ hour school day on 3 different days. All probes revealed zero instances of the target behaviors, indicating generalization effects across time and settings.

These results are interesting in that the self-management procedures represented the only intervention used. Morrow and Presswood (1984) speculated that the rapid and marked changes in the student's behavior resulted in more social interactions and approval from peers and adults. Additionally, the inclusion of self-monitoring, self-evaluation, and self-recording may also have prompted a self-reinforcement reaction. Advantages of these procedures include its (a) ease of implementation by paraprofessionals, (b) cost effectiveness, as no backup reinforcers were required, and (c) flexibility of application to a number of ongoing classroom instructional activities.

Multiple Agitated/Disruptive Behaviors.   In a series of three studies, Gardner and colleagues (Cole et al., 1985; Gardner, Clees, & Cole, 1983; Gardner, Cole, Berry, & Nowinski, 1983) evaluated the effects of a treatment package that included multiple self-management procedures. Subjects in the studies were adults with mild to moderate levels of mental retardation who displayed chronic problems that had not responded to a variety of psychological, psychiatric, and behavioral procedures. The program rationale and procedures were based on the authors' clinical experiences with clients who presented such chronic difficulties as verbal and physical aggression, temper outbursts, inappropriate expression of anger, and other states of heightened negative emotional arousal that suggested that these clients often acted impulsively in response to sources of provocation. The clients provided minimal if any indication that they engaged in the self-management activities of self-observation, self-evaluation, self-instruction, or self-consequation, or that such skills were in their repertoires.

In the initial study, Gardner, Cole et al. (1983) evaluated the effects of a self-management package on the high rate disruptive verbal behaviors (e.g., teasing and taunting, swearing, name calling, threatening, yelling) of two adults with moderate mental retardation who attended a vocational training program. In the absence of frequent staff intervention, the disruptive verbal behaviors typically escalated into acts of physical aggression.

Both clients had been enrolled in a vocational training program prior to the study but were irregular in attendance and erratic in work production, and demonstrated highly disruptive social behaviors. Both had experienced lengthy suspensions from work because of staff difficulties in managing their behaviors.

During initial baseline conditions, clients received social praise and monetary reinforcers on a variable interval 3-minute schedule. Reinforcement was contingent on such appropriate work and social behaviors as displaying positive affect, being on task, working quietly, ignoring provocative behaviors of peers, and fulfilling staff requests. Following baseline, self-management training was provided, initially in a training room and later in the work setting for *in vivo* rehearsal.

During a 1-day training session, each client was initially taught to:

1. *Self monitor* (discriminate the occurrence of such behaviors as yelling/not yelling, teasing/not teasing, and singing loudly/working quietly. Following trainer modeling and appropriate client labeling of the behaviors, the client was guided to self-monitor his or her own role-played behaviors.

2. *Self-evaluate* his or her own actions. Appropriate behaviors were labeled by the trainer as "good adult worker" behavior and undesirable behaviors were labeled "not adult worker" behavior. Numerous problem situations were described and modeled, the client prompted to role play appropriate and inappropriate responses to each and to self-evaluate these actions. In addition, each client was provided a laminated 6 × 8½ inch card displayed at the work station. A colored photograph of the client smiling was attached to one side and was labeled as "good adult worker," while the flip side, with a photograph of the client frowning, was labeled as "not adult worker" behavior.

   Several opportunities for role playing various behaviors were provided with the client intermittently labeling his or her own behavior (self-monitoring) and, using the display card, assessing it as "good adult worker" behavior or "not adult worker" behavior (self-evaluation). Finally, each client was prompted to rehearse several prosocial alternatives to inappropriate behaviors, using self-instruction when appropriate.

3. *Self-consequate* his or her own behavior (i.e., to self-deliver a reinforcer or to self-punish with a brief timeout and response cost contingent on self-evaluation of behavior). The trainer, removing a coin from a container placed on the client's work table, clipped it to the good adult worker side of the display card. The card was flipped several times to emphasize that "good adult worker" behavior earned money, while "not adult worker" behavior does not.

Finally, each client was provided a timer, taught to set it independently for a designated period of time, and informed, "Whenever you decide to be a "good adult worker" until the bell rings, you'll earn a coin." The trainer initially modeled setting the timer and differentially consequating behaviors. When appropriate behavior was engaged in throughout the time interval, the client was prompted to (a) self-monitor, (b) self-evaluate, and (c) self-reinforce by taking a coin from the card. In contrast, inappropriate behavior was followed by immediate flipping of the display card to the "not adult worker" picture and stopping the timer. Inappropriate behavior thus was followed by a self-initiated timeout (i.e., temporary loss of opportunity to work and earn money) and a response cost (i.e., loss of minutes accumulated prior to occurrence of the inappropriate behavior). The client was prompted to rehearse, with the trainer, alternative appropriate behaviors and, when the client decided that he or she was ready to begin working again, to flip over the card to the "good adult worker" picture, reset the timer, and begin working. Each client then rehearsed engaging in and labeling the entire behavior-consequence contingency.

On resuming work in the workshop, clients were provided additional training to insure generalization to this setting. Whenever inappropriate behavior occurred, the trainer prompted the client through the above-described sequence, correcting errors and labeling and praising appropriate responses. Because *in vivo* events such as a threatening gesture from a peer frequently preceded inappropriate behavior, these peer interactions served as a basis for rehearsal of alternative self-managed behaviors. Whenever possible, the peer(s) who provoked the client participated with the client in rehearsal of more appropriate behaviors.

During the initial self-management phase, the trainer continued to verbally prompt the client upon hesitation (e.g., to set the timer) or error (e.g., failing to attach a coin to the display card) in the behavior sequence. Staff also intervened at the end of each successfully completed work interval and upon every occurrence of inappropriate behavior. The client was prompted to self-monitor, self-evaluate, and self-consequate and to rehearse appropriate alternative behaviors following inappropriate ones. Trainer intervention was faded gradually as each client demonstrated independence in the various self-management activities.

A combined reversal and modified changing criterion design was used to assess the intervention package. An immediate and significant reduction in the disruptive verbalizations was obtained for both clients. Treatment gains were maintained during a fading phase and at 6-month followup.

In a second investigation of this treatment package, Gardner, Clees et al. (1983) assessed its effects on the high rate disruptive vocalizations (verbal ruminations and nonspeech sounds) of a man who had moderate mental retardation in a vocational training setting. These behaviors seemed to be self-stimulatory in nature and unrelated to current external stimulation. Although not directed toward others initially, the content, frequency, and volume of these verbal behaviors resulted in agitated/disruptive reactions from peers that required staff intervention. A combined treatment withdrawal and modified changing criterion design was used to evaluate treatment effects. In addition, potential concurrent changes in behaviors (talking to others, stereotypic/motoric movements, and production rate) not selected as specific targets of intervention were evaluated.

Disruptive vocalizations showed an immediate effect upon introduction of treatment (97.5% to near-zero occurrence following 3 weeks of treatment). The near-zero level was maintained through fading and at 6- and 12-month followup. Similar therapeutic effects were obtained for collateral behaviors not targeted for intervention. Stereotyped behaviors were virtually eliminated, production rate increased, and appropriate talking to others improved.

In the third study in this series, Cole et al. (1985) evaluated the effects of the treatment program on the high rate disruptive behaviors of six adults functioning in the mild to moderate range of mental retardation. All clients displayed chronic and severe behavioral/emotional difficulties. Although each had been provided a range of psychiatric and psychological treatment, none had demonstrated desired progress. In fact, for all subjects, clinically significant conduct difficulties had resulted in dismissal from, or precluded placement in, community vocational rehabilitation programs.

Disruptive verbal and physical behaviors specific to each subject served as treatment targets. In addition to the training program described previously, clients in this study were provided more detailed self-instructional training. Video and audio tapes of specific provocative situations (e.g., peer taunting, staff corrective feedback) were presented. The trainer modeled appropriate self-verbalizations in the presence of these provocative cues (e.g., "Jerry's teasing me, but I won't yell. I'm a good adult worker, I'll ignore him."). Later, the client was prompted to use these statements to self-direct his or her appropriate behavior. During client rehearsal, the duration and intensity of the simulated provocation was gradually increased and the client was encouraged to speak more and more softly, with the ultimate goal of subvocal self-talk under actual provocation. Following individual training, each client resumed working in the vocational training setting with the program materials placed at his or her work station. In addition to the *in vivo* training procedures previously described, each client was frequently encouraged to self-instruct and rehearse appropriate coping responses.

A combined treatment withdrawal and multiple baseline design was used to assess treatment effects. The intervention package produced immediate and clinically significant reductions in severe conduct difficulties in all six clients. Nine-month followup under different work conditions revealed continued maintenance of treatment gains.

Self-Management: Maintenance Strategy

Robertson, Simon, Pachman, and Drabman (1979) demonstrated the value of self-management procedures in maintaining positive behavioral gains obtained under externally managed procedures. Subjects consisted of a special education class of 12 children, 5 to 11 years of age, who were in the moderate to mild range of mental retardation. The children were described as demonstrating a high level of classroom disruptiveness.

Following a baseline period, the teacher initially set a timer for five consecutive 10-minute periods during the morning classroom session. When the timer sounded, the teacher moved around the room and told each child whether he or she had been "good," "okay," or "not good" during the preceding period. Each child was informed of the reasons for his or her rating. This continued for 17 days. During a token reinforcement phase that followed, the children were awarded points on the basis of the teacher ratings. Points were exchangeable daily for edibles and/or special activities.

Following 12 days of the token program, the children were informed that they would rate themselves and attempt to match the teacher ratings. A bonus was awarded for matches and a penalty was imposed for failure to match. After the class had demonstrated proficiency in matching the teacher's ratings (24 days), the matching requirements were gradually faded (28 days). Next, the children monitored themselves independently and points were awarded based on each child's self-ratings. Points were exchangeable for backup reinforcers. Use of points was faded and baseline conditions reinstated.

Teacher feedback produced a substantial reduction in disruptive behaviors. Further reduction was noted following introduction of tokens and matching. These low levels were maintained throughout the fading, self-evaluation, and return to baseline phases. Thus, the children's self-evaluations were functional in maintaining the treatment effects obtained by teacher evaluation and token reinforcement. Of interest was the finding that these results generalized to an afternoon period during which no treatment was provided. Additionally, high agreement was obtained between teacher ratings and student ratings, even in phases during which the children were unaware that they were being rated by the teacher.

CONCLUSIONS

As is evident, the empirical literature devoted to use of self-management procedures in treatment of severe aberrant behaviors displayed by those with mental retardation is quite limited. The limitation is evident both in the small number of studies available and in the small sample sizes and restrictions in the diversity of severity and types of problem behaviors treated. Further, while the literature is suggestive of potential therapeutic applicability, the demonstration of independent contributions of specific self-management components is lacking. In most studies, the self-management procedures were embedded with external procedures in a more comprehensive program. For example, while self-reinforcement procedures were present in some studies, these did not meet the criteria of independent self-reinforcement. As defined by Bandura (1976), self-reinforcement involves three conditions, namely (a) free access to reinforcers, (b) a self-imposed standard of performance that one is to attain prior to reinforcing oneself, and (c) the self-determination that the performance criterion has been satisfied prior to reinforcing oneself. In the studies reported in which self-reinforcement was included, the person did not have free access to reinforcers and the performance standards were set by external agents.

Despite these limitations, the results of these initial studies are encouraging. Clients were able to discriminate the attainment of performance standards and, based on this observation, to self-deliver reinforcers made available to them. Other more cognitively limited clients were able to self-monitor their own behaviors and, as a result, to reduce the occurrence of their problems. The shift from external control toward self-management illustrated in these studies represents a major departure from the external behavior therapy practices of the past.

REFERENCES

Agran, M., & Martin, J. E. (1987). Applying a technology of self-control in community environments for individuals who are mentally retarded. In M. Hersen, R. M. Eisler, & P. M. Miller (Eds.), *Progress in behavior modification* (Vol. 21, pp. 108–151). New York: Academic Press.

Alberto, P. A., Sharpton, W. R., Briggs, A., & Stright, M. H. (1986). Facilitating task acquisition through the use of a self-operated auditory prompting system. *Journal of the Association for Persons with Severe Handicaps, 11,* 85–91.

Axelrod, S. (1987). Functional and structural analyses of behavior: Approaches leading to reduced use of punishment procedures? *Research in Developmental Disabilities, 8,* 165–178.

Bandura, A. (1976). Self-reinforcement: Theoretical and methodological considerations. *Behaviorism, 4,* 135–155.

Berkowitz, A. J. (1987). The AAMD position statement on aversive therapy. *Mental Retardation, 25,* 118.

Bornstein, P. H., Bach, P. J., & Anton, B. (1982). Behavioral treatment of psychopathological disorders. In J. L. Matson & R. P. Barrett (Eds.), *Psychopathology of the mentally retarded.* New York: Grune & Stratton.

Carr, E. G., & Durand, V. M. (1985). Reducing behavior problems through functional communication training. *Journal of Applied Behavior Analysis, 18,* 111–126.

Carr, E. G., & Newsom, C. (1985). Demand-related tantrums: Conceptualization and treatment. *Behavior Modification, 9,* 403–426.

Carr, E. G., Newsom, C., & Binkoff, J. A. (1980). Escape as a factor in the aggressive behavior of two retarded children. *Journal of Applied Behavior Analysis, 13,* 101–117.

Cole, C. L., Gardner, W. I., & Karan, O. C. (1985). Self-management training of mentally retarded adults presenting severe conduct difficulties. *Applied Research in Mental Retardation, 6,* 337–347.

Durand, V. M., & Carr, E. G. (1987). Social influences on "self-stimulatory" behaviors: Analysis and treatment applications. *Journal of Applied Behavior Analysis, 20,* 119–132.

Foxx, R. M., McMorrow, M. J., Bittle, R. G., & Bechtel, D. R. (1986). The successful treatment of a dually-diagnosed deaf man's aggression with a program that included contingent electric shock. *Behavior Therapy, 17,* 170–186.

Gardner, W. I. (1988). Behavior therapies: Past, present, future. In J. Stark, F. Menolascino, M. Albarelli, & V. Gray (Eds.), *Mental retardation and mental health: Classification, diagnosis, treatment, services* (pp. 161–172). New York: Springer-Verlag.

Gardner, W. I., Clees, T. J., & Cole, C. L. (1983). Self-management of disruptive verbal ruminations by a mentally retarded adult. *Applied Research in Mental Retardation, 4,* 41–58.

Gardner, W. I., & Cole, C. L. (1984). Aggression and related conduct difficulties in the mentally retarded: A multicomponent behavior model. In S. E. Bruening, J. L. Matson, & R. P. Barrett (Eds.), *Advances in mental retardation and developmental disabilities: A research annual* (Vol. 2, pp. 41–84). Greenwich, CT: JAI Press.

Gardner, W. I., & Cole, C. L. (1985). Acting-out disorders. In M. Hersen (Ed.), *Practice of inpatient behavior therapy: A clinical guide* (pp. 203–230). New York: Grune & Stratton.

Gardner, W. I., & Cole, C. L. (1987). Managing aggressive behavior: A behavioral diagnostic approach. *Psychiatric Aspects of Mental Retardation Reviews, 6,* 21–25.

Gardner, W. I., & Cole, C. L. (1988). Self-monitoring. In E. S. Shapiro & T. R. Kratochwill (Eds.), *Behavioral assessment in schools: Conceptual foundations and practical applications* (pp. 206–246). New York: Guilford Press.

Gardner, W. I., & Cole, C. L. (in press). Aggression and related conduct difficulties: A behavior diagnostic and treatment model. In J. L. Matson (Ed.), *Handbook of behavior modification with persons with mental retardation* (Rev. Ed.) New York: Plenum Press.

Gardner, W. I., Cole, C. L., Berry, D. L., & Nowinski, J. M. (1983). Reduction of disruptive behaviors in mentally retarded adults: A self-management approach. *Behavior Modification, 7,* 76–96.

Guess, D., Helmstetter, E., Turnbull, H. R., & Knowlton, S. (1987). Use of aversive procedures with persons who are disabled: An historical review and critical analysis. *Monograph of the Association for Persons with Severe Handicaps, 2*(1).

Matson, J. L., & Andrasik, F. (1982). Training leisure-time social-interaction skills to mentally retarded adults. *American Journal of Mental Deficiency, 86,* 533–542.

McNally, R. J., Kompik, J. J., & Sherman, G. (1984). Increasing the productivity of mentally retarded workers through self-management. *Analysis and Intervention in Developmental Disabilities, 4,* 129–135.

Morrow, L. W., & Presswood, S. (1984). The effects of a self-control technique on eliminating three stereotypic behaviors in a multiply-handicapped institutionalized adolescent. *Behavior Disorders, 9,* 247–253.

Reese, R. M., Sherman, J. A., & Sheldon, J. (1984). Reducing agitated-disruptive behavior of mentally retarded residents of community group homes: The role of self-recording and peer-prompted self-recording. *Analysis and Intervention in Developmental Disabilities, 4,* 91–107.

Repp, A. C., & Brulle, A. R. (1981). Reducing aggressive behavior of mentally retarded persons. In J. L. Matson & J. R. McCartney (Eds.), *Handbook of behavior modification with the mentally retarded* (pp. 177–210). New York: Plenum Press.

Robertson, S. J., Simon, S. J., Pachman, J. S., & Drabman, R. S. (1979). Self-control and generalization procedures in a classroom of disruptive retarded children. *Child Behavior Therapy, 1,* 347–362.

Rolider, A., & Van Houten, R. (1985). Movement suppression time-out for undesirable behavior in psychotic and severely developmentally delayed children. *Journal of Applied Behavior Analysis, 18,* 275–288.

Rosine, L. P. C., & Martin, G. L. (1983). Self-management training to decrease undesirable behavior of mentally handicapped adults. *Rehabilitation Psychology, 28,* 195–205.

Shapiro, E. S. (1981). Self-control procedures with the mentally retarded. In M. Hersen, R. M. Eisler, & P. M. Miller (Eds.), *Progress in behavior modification* (Vol. 12, pp. 265–297). New York: Academic Press.

Shapiro, E. S. (1986). Behavior modification: Self-control and cognitive procedures. In R. P. Barrett (Ed.), *Severe behavior disorders in the mentally retarded* (pp. 61–97). New York: Plenum.

Shapiro, E. S., Browder, D. M., & D'Huyvetters, K. L. (1984). Increasing academic productivity of severely multi-handicapped children with self-management: Idiosyncratic effects. *Analysis and Intervention in Developmental Disabilities, 4,* 171–188.

Zegiob, L., Klukas, N., & Junginger, J. (1978). Reactivity of self-monitoring procedures with retarded adolescents. *American Journal of Mental Deficiency, 83,* 156–163.

Punishment for People With Developmental Disabilities

Floyd O'Brien
University of the Pacific

THE MISUNDERSTANDING OF PUNISHMENT

Some people with developmental disabilities thwart attempts at normalization by performing maladaptive behaviors (e.g., aggression, property destruction, and self-injurious behavior). They may misbehave even when adequate positive reinforcement is available for adaptive skills (cf., Matson & DiLorenzo, 1984; O'Brien, 1981; Risley, 1968). Typically, public agencies (e.g., departments of education, developmental disabilities, and social services) purport to serve in maximizing normalization—develop as normal behavior as possible within settings and with procedures as normal as possible (Wolfensberger, 1972). Yet, these same agencies often establish regulations (i.e., restrictions) on the use of punishment in manners that retard normalization. Students are transferred to classrooms further from mainstream education when teachers are disallowed the use of punishment. Residents of community care homes are transferred to hospitals when the use of punishment is disallowed, or when it becomes too costly to obtain permission to use it. Typically, such regulations stem from a misunderstanding of the term *punishment.*

Dictionaries exemplify the misunderstanding of punishment. In *Webster's Ninth New Collegiate Dictionary* (1987), for example, we find terms like "suffering," "pain," "inflicted on an offender," and "severe, rough, or disastrous treatment" within the definition of *punishment.* That public agencies regulate such treatment is laudable; yet pain, suffering, and disastrous treatment are more indicative of neglect than of the use of punishment. A resident of a nursing home who blinded himself by gouging his eyes, destroyed countless brain cells by banging his head, and lost several fingers by chewing them has experienced pain and suffering. His treatment could be described as disastrous. The disastrous treatment, however, is caused not by the use of punishment, but by its neglect. Had punishment been applied, the needless pain could have been stopped. Thus, although support should be given the public in attempts at regulating against disastrous treatment, support should be withheld for any regulation of punishment that serves to thwart its appropriate use.

The transdisciplinary team is usually the first line of defense against disastrous treatment. Typically, such teams consist of a client, a case manager, a teacher, a psychologist, and a parent. The teams prescribe the services the clients receive, establish goals, and review the efficacy of the treatments. As such these teams are the most valid sources of information about the clients, the services they receive, the history of treatments, placements, and so forth.

It seems curious that these teams are often the ones that note the need for using "therapeutic punishment" (Matson & DiLorenzo, 1984), prescribe it, and then are disallowed its use by some bureaucratic entity that has no current knowledge of the client. Sometimes, this entity might be the principal of a school, a regulator from the department that licenses the care home, or a regulator from an agency that coordinates programs for people with disabilities. Purportedly to regulate against abuse, these entities restrict the teams from prescribing punishment. In the process, such entities further exacerbate the greatest abuse of people with disabilities in the nation—not providing them the services they need.

DEFINITION OF PUNISHMENT

In 1966, Azrin and Holz provided a functional definition of *punishment*. Their definition presents the phenomenon of punishment as a direct relationship between behavior and the environment. They posited that punishment is a reduction in the future probability of a behavior resulting from providing a consequence for that behavior. The consequence was called a *punishing stimulus* or a *punisher* and was defined as a consequence for a behavior that reduces the future probability of that behavior (response).

Although this definition will be adhered to throughout the chapter, some prefer to include the functional relationship in the definition of the consequence (punishing stimulus or punisher) and to limit the definition of the procedure to an operational one. Thus, *punishment* is the delivery of a punisher for a behavior and a *punisher* is an environmental event (stimulus) that reduces the future probability of the behavior it follows (cf., Morse & Kelleher, 1977). Regardless, the perspective of punishment's definition in the functional, direct manner has become so popular that this perspective is the prominent one today (cf., Axelrod & Apsche, 1983; Johnston, 1972; Matson & DiLorenzo, 1984; Morse & Kelleher, 1977).

This direct definition of punishment, then, includes only a reduction in a behavior resulting from a punisher being provided as a consequence for that behavior. No "pain," "trauma," "unpleasantness," or "annoyance" is required. Thus, when a consequence for a behavior results in one's decreasing the behavior, that is *punishment*, even when the person whose behavior is being punished admits that it is not unpleasant, painful, annoying, and so forth.

For example, O'Brien and Azrin (1970) tested a gadget that provided a vibrating stimulus on a shoulder when a person slouched. With a description of what the gadget did, all people who were tested slouched less when the vibrator was operative than when it was disconnected. In this study, the feedback reduced the frequency of slouching and therefore served as a punisher. Yet, the opposite effect occurred when people were asked to slouch as much as possible (i.e., they slouched more when the vibrator was operative than when it was disconnected). Thus, the same stimulus was a punisher for a behavior under one condition and a reinforcer for the same behavior under the other condition. The point is that the stimulus was reported to be benign—not annoying, painful, or noxious. Thus, punishment may occur even when there is nothing traumatic, annoying, or objectionable in the treatment. Because that is so, it is fallacious to argue against using punishment based on the notion that it must be painful and annoying.

AT RISK METHODS
CONFUSED WITH PUNISHMENT

Another source of the misunderstanding of punishment is its inclusion with other treatments that have high risk potentials for producing problems. In the 1950s and '60s, for example, electroconvulsive shock therapy was provided in a manner that caused brain damage and other injury (Torrey, 1983). Soon thereafter, some authors (e.g., Lovas & Simmons, 1969; and Risley, 1968) reported using contingent electric shock to reduce self-injurious and self-stimulatory behaviors within the punishment paradigm. Although contingent electric shock was painful, it was provided immediately after the misbehavior, lasted only a second or two, and produced no physical damage (Carr & Lovaas, 1983). As such, contingent electric shock had no serious risks, but was classed with electroconvulsive shock therapy (an intervention of high risk). And worse, because contingent electric shock was punishment, punishment, itself, was misunderstood to be an "at risk" procedure.

Two other medical interventions used to change behavior were erroneously called "behavior modification" and are "at risk" interventions. One of them is surgery of the brain (Torrey, 1983); suffice it to say that all surgery has risks. The other medical intervention is chemotherapy, sometimes referred to in the perjorative as "chemical restraint." The drugs typically used in this intervention have short-term and long-term side effects:

extrapyramidal symptoms are examples of the former; tardive dyskinesia, the latter (Davis & Gierl, 1984). Thus, these interventions are provided "at risk." Yet, they should not be classed with "behavior modification," and their "at risk" character has nothing to do with the use of therapeutic punishment.

Solitary confinement, physical restraint, and deprivation have been used in penal and treatment institutions and were often called "punishment" (Alexander & Selesnick, 1966). This set the occasion for their being confused with therapeutic punishment techniques. Punishment in a time-out room for 10 minutes was confused with solitary confinement in prison, for example; or, punishment by restraining a client's arm for 10 seconds was confused with restraining a person to bed with soft ties for days, and deprivation by giving one cup of water and one plate of cereal a day to a prisoner was likened to punishment by removing a client's tray of food for 30 seconds for a misbehavior during a meal. The confusion of these procedures with therapeutic punishment furthers the misunderstanding of punishment.

Many would consider these procedures of the correction and treatment institutions to be cruel when treating people with developmental disabilities, and would probably do whatever became necessary to assure that clients never receive such disastrous treatment. But to equate these with the punishment procedures noted above is faulty. The former are cruel; the latter are therapeutic and essentially risk free. Nonetheless, regulators typically restrain both without prior approval and require similar prior reviews to use either, presumably based on the misunderstanding that the two are of the same class.

PUNISHMENT THAT
IS NORMAL

Behavior analysts no more invented the laws of behavior than physicists invented the laws of nature. Both describe the normal universe; neither invented it. And like the physicist who bemoans the fact that sunlight includes harmful rays, a behavior analyst may bemoan the fact that punishment exists or, more accurately, that pain, discomfort, annoyance, and the like are normally present in our universe. Environmental events (stimuli) associated with these states often serve as punishers in many behavior patterns that would produce damage to our bodies. Putting pencils in our ears, walking through solid objects, climbing trees during thunderstorms, cramming metal clothes hangers into electric outlets, remaining in sub-zero temperatures for long periods, and so forth are behaviors reduced by punishers to the betterment of ourselves and our species.

People too have long used punishment before behavior analysts studied it, and they continue doing so. Teachers and parents use corporal punishment (shaking and spanking); police use restraint (handcuffs); parents take away toys from children misusing them; preachers require penance, condemn to damnation, or exclude from the church; courts fine and imprison people; schools use detention, exclusion, and expulsion; and we all experience verbal abuse, criticism, denial, and so forth in normal social interactions with one another (cf., Franks, 1984; Kazdin, 1975). Thus, punishment is normal within the physical and social realms, so normal that the public hysteria regarding its use in therapy seems irrational.

LABORATORY RESEARCH
ON PUNISHMENT

In reviews of laboratory research on punishment (e.g., Matson & Di-Lorenzo, 1984; Van Houten, 1983), authors typically devote most attention to the review by Azrin and Holz (1966) and their concluding 14 recommendations for maximizing the effects of punishment. For the purpose of this chapter, it is unnecessary to review this voluminous literature, nor would space allow it. Suffice it to say that there is a rich source of scientific literature on punishment, and that they are in error who restrict punishment from their therapeutic options on the basis of inadequate research.

Of the 14 recommendations mentioned above, most are of utmost concern when using punishment in treatment. For example, any environmental events that serve to strengthen the punished behavior should be eliminated or reduced (e.g., establishing operations, discriminative stimuli, and reinforcers). Unauthorized escape from punishment should be disallowed. Alternative behaviors should be established and richly reinforced. The punisher should be delivered at a high intensity (never increased progressively from lower intensities), paired with no reinforcement for the punished behavior, delivered immediately, and delivered for every instance of the punished behavior (Azrin and Holz, 1966).

Although no more laboratory research will be discussed in this chapter, readers are encouraged to review the literature and should certainly do so if they are considering the use of therapeutic punishment in their practice. Any of the three reviews mentioned in the first paragraph of this section would serve.

TYPES OF PUNISHMENT

When authors present reviews of punishment techniques, they typically emphasize the type of behavior, the consequence provided as a punisher, and the effects on the frequency of that behavior. Before doing so, however, this author feels compelled to remind the reader of the relativity of consequences to antecedents (cf., Van Houten, 1983). This may be necessary to avert the readers' failure in applying techniques discussed for similar behaviors of people with dissimilar antecedents. For example, the gadget applied for slouching and discussed earlier (O'Brien & Azrin, 1970) resulted in more slouching when people were asked to slouch and reduced slouching without this antecedent. Thus, if one applied this technique to reduce the slouching of a client who was previously told to slouch as much as possible, the treatment would fail. In this example, the consequence functions as a punisher without antecedent instructions to slouch, but as a reinforcer with that antecedent. This exemplifies the relativity between consequences and antecedents to which readers must remain alert when reading reviews that discuss consequences but provide inadequate descriptions of antecedents.

Michael (1982) separated these antecedents into classes. He named those antecedents that effect whether the consequence is a punisher, a reinforcer, or neutral as establishing operations. The instruction to slouch mentioned above is an establishing operation. Deprivation/satiation of reinforcers is another. For example, providing candy may be a reinforcer if the client has been without food for 2 hours, neutral if the client has just eaten enough candy, and a punisher if so much candy has already been eaten that the client is nauseous. Time-out may be reinforcing for a client who is fatigued, a squirt of lemon juice into the mouth may be reinforcing if the client has been without liquids for a long time, and manual restraint by a caregiver may be reinforcing if the client has been without human attention for hours.

Another class of antecedents Michael (1982) named *discriminative.* Of most importance in this chapter are antecedents that may have established punishers as discriminative stimuli, events that set the occasion for a behavior's reinforcement. For example, clients' signing for something may be reinforced only if caregivers are attending to them. In this case, caregivers' attention is a discriminative stimulus for signing. As such, behaviors that result in attention may be reinforced. Given a plan that directs caregivers to restrain clients' hands for 3 seconds after they slap themselves, slapping may be reinforced by the attention it produces if clients then sign for and receive what they wanted (e.g., a drink, being taken to the toilet, or having a radio turned on). Consequences for maladaptive behaviors must always be analyzed as to their possible discriminative functions lest punishers serve as discriminative stimuli, and thereby reinforce the maladaptive behavior supposedly being punished.

From a general perspective, there are two types of punishment: giving a punisher for a behavior and removing a reinforcer for a behavior. Unfortunately, it is often difficult to distinguish between them (e.g., Is sending the child to her room punishment because being alone in her room is a punisher she has been given or because reinforcers outside of her room are being taken from her?). Also, punishment often consists of more than one of each process (e.g., reprimand, removal of a reinforcer, and requiring an apology). This state of affairs disallows us from using that general classification. Thus, the names that are most prevalent in the literature are used in this chapter.

Reprimands

Van Houten and Doleys (1983) defined reprimands as "expressions of disapproval" (p. 46). This definition allows for many forms, including gestures, frowns, and soft or loud volume utterances. These authors reviewed several studies that recorded the frequency of reprimands used by parents in homes and teachers in classrooms. The findings ranged from about 11 to 35 an hour. These numbers tend to confirm the notion that verbal reprimand is the most used type of punishment.

Six people with developmental disabilities substantially decreased their body rocking when researchers yelled "Stop rocking!" immediately after they began doing so (Baumeister & Forehand, 1972). A preschool-aged child with mental retardation reduced throwing objects when the researchers reprimanded the child for throwing (Sajwaj, Culver, Hall, & Lehr, 1972). Schutz, Wehman, Renzaglia, and Karan (1978) demonstrated that reprimands reduced misbehaviors by adults in a workshop, and Jones and Miller (1974) showed that reprimands reduced misbehaviors by students in classrooms. Finally, a child with mental retardation suppressed pinching and biting herself when teachers pointed at her while shouting "No!" as a consequence (Hall et al., 1971).

These studies demonstrate that reprimands may serve as punishers to decrease maladaptive behaviors performed by people with developmental disabilities. In many other studies (e.g., Henricksen & Doughty, 1967; O'Brien & Azrin, 1972; Repp, Deitz, & Speir, 1974; Van Houten & Doleys, 1983), reprimands served as components in punishment techniques that included other procedures. However, these studies disallow readers from separating the additive effect, if any, of the reprimands from the other components of the punishment techniques. Also, most studies disallow readers from a finer analysis of the many parameters included in the reprimand. These parameters include how close the reprimander was to the client, whether eye contact was provided and for how long contact was maintained, how loud the voice was, how explicit the content of the reprimand was, and so forth. Fortunately, some researchers are investigating these parameters (e.g., Abramowitz & O'Leary, 1987), and Van Houten and Doleys (1983) discussed some studies showing that eye contact, grasping (or shaking) the client while reprimanding, and being closer to the client increased the efficacy of reprimands. We join these authors in recommending more such studies and in deploring the paucity of research on this most often used type of punishment.

Time-out

Another often used type of punishment is time-out, originally named "time-out from positive reinforcement" (Ferster & Skinner, 1957). Although the term has been applied to many different procedures, and different authors have provided variant definitions (Matson & DiLorenzo, 1984), the one adhered to in this chapter is by Brantner and Doherty (1983): ". . . a period of time in a less reinforcing environment made contingent on a behavior" (p. 87). By emphasizing a time period, this definition tends to highlight the essential difference between time-out and other procedures that include less reinforcement (e.g., extinction and response cost). Also, this definition alerts the reader directly to the relativity between antecedent and consequence, a concern discussed earlier regarding all punishment, and one that is most crucial in the many procedures called time-out.

The period of time in which less reinforcement is available can be provided in infinite ways. The least intrusive types are classified as *nonexclusion time-out* and involve the least amount of restriction from the ongoing activity. For example, Risley and Wolf (1967) timed-out children for misbehaviors during one-on-one language training by simply looking away from the children for a few seconds. During those few seconds, the training activity ceased. Porterfield, Herbert-Jackson, and Risley (1976) introduced a time-out technique that continued the training activity but excluded the misbehaver for the time-out period. They provided this *contingent observation* period by moving the misbehaver's chair a little away from the periphery of the activity for a period of time, during which the student could observe the training activity being provided to other students but remained inactive in the instruction. Foxx and Shapiro (1978) provided a similar nonexclusion time-out by having the students wear ribbons during time-in. Immediately after a student misbehaved, the ribbon was removed, and the student was ignored during the time-out period. O'Brien and Azrin (1972) and Augustine and Cipani (1982) reduced misbehaviors during mealtimes by removing the diner's tray of food for a short period, during which the diner remained seated and observed others eating.

Facial screening is another type of time-out that leaves the misbehaver at the site of the activity. In this type of time-out, researchers cover misbehavers' faces with cloth during the period. People with developmental disabilities have learned to decrease self-stimulatory, self-injurious, out-of-seat, and disruptive behaviors with facial screening (Lutzker, 1978; Spencer & Lutzker, 1974; Zegiob, Jenkins, Becker, & Bristow, 1976).

Somewhat more restrictive types of time-out are called *exclusion time-out* and involve removing the misbehavers from the site of the activity, but not isolating them (Brantner & Doherty, 1983). For example, Bostow and Bailey (1969) reduced disruptive and aggressive behaviors of an institutionalized client by requiring the client to remain in a corner for a couple of minutes as a consequence. Barrett (1969) and Hobbs, Forehand, and Murray (1978) also used standing in the corner. Carlson, Arnold, Becker, and Madsen (1968) used a time-out chair.

The most restrictive type of time-out is called *seclusion* (May et al., 1975) or *isolation* (Brantner & Doherty, 1983) *time-out.* In this method, the client is placed in a separate area, usually a room, typically devoid of other people and objects that may be reinforcing. An early example of isolation time-out concerned reducing a child's tantrums, self-injurious behaviors, and throwing his glasses by sending him to his room for 10 minutes as a consequence (Wolf, Risley, & Mees, 1964). Another example is Webster and Azrin's (1973) *required relaxation.* In this study, institutionalized people with developmental disabilities were required to bed rest for a period of time following agitated/disruptive behaviors. Finally, Hamilton, Stephens, and Allen (1967) decreased misbehaviors in women with mental retardation by requiring their confinement in a time-out area as a consequence.

In part, these categories of time-out were chosen because of their prominence in other reviews (cf., Brantner & Doherty, 1983; Matson & DiLorenzo, 1984). As Matson and DiLorenzo (1984) implied, the categories involve separation on at least three variables: removal of the misbehaver, removal of the reinforcer, and the amount of reinforcement sources removed (e.g., removal of a food tray vs. isolation in a barren room). Thus, exact categorization is unachievable.

As noted, the complexity of categorization is created by the number of parameters on which different time-out techniques may vary. In the reviews mentioned above, these parameters included (a) duration; (b) types of prompt to enter time-out (e.g., none, verbal, and physical); (c) location; (d) whether a stimulus was provided to identify onset or termination of the time-out period; (e) the schedule (continuous or intermittent) of time-out administration; (f) whether exit from time-out was contingent on behavior, time, or both; (g) whether a warning was given before time-out was applied; (h) the type of explanation, if any, given to the offender when time-out was administered; and (i) the relative reinforcement of the time-in activity. How these parameters influence the efficacy of time-out is discussed in the reviews mentioned (Brantner & Dougherty, 1983; Matson &

DiLorenzo, 1984), and readers are referred to them for more elaborate discussions.

Although a few studies have reported ineffective time-out techniques for people with developmental disabilities (e.g., Harris & Wolchik, 1979), many others report effective treatments for problems like misbehaviors at meals, noncompliance, self-stimulatory behavior, aggression, property destruction, errors in instruction, faking convulsions (seizures), tantrums, elective mutism, self-injurious behaviors, and perseverative/echolalic speech (Brantner & Doherty, 1983; Cipani, 1981; Matson & DiLorenzo, 1984; O'Brien, 1981; Repp & Brulle, 1981; Schroeder, Schroeder, Rojahn, & Mulick, 1981).

Physical Restraint

As with other punishment procedures, it is difficult to classify physical restraint. Is being restrained from movement a punisher because it is a punisher in and of itself, because it restricts the person from other reinforcers, or both? Matson and DiLorenzo (1984), for example, classified physical restraint as a special type of time-out. The reader may note that it does fit the definition of time-out used in this chapter. However, restraint is such a special type of time-out that it justifies a section unto itself.

Matson and DiLorenzo (1984) defined physical restraint more generally than do the medically oriented authors who described restraint with leather or soft-ties of body parts, usually to beds, to prevent clients from injuring themselves. Matson and DiLorenzo included any physical restriction of movement of limbs when used as a consequence of behavior as physical restraint. However, they also indicated that it be for a specified time period. This qualifier would dismiss from the category of physical restraint those techniques involving restraint of a limb until a behavioral criterion is met. Thus, this chapter adheres to the Matson and DiLorenzo definition without the temporal qualifier.

Very restrictive body restraints have typically been used to treat self-injurious behaviors (Baumeister & Rollings, 1976). Hamilton, Stephens, and Allen (1967) reduced headbanging with contingent physical restraint, and Bucher, Reykdal, and Albin (1976) reduced pica. Cipani and Wolter (1983) used brief physical restraint to decrease self-injurious behavior of a young adult with profound mental retardation. In teaching relaxation skills to clients who engaged in self-injurious behaviors, Schroeder, Peterson, Solomon, and Artley (1977) provided and removed manual restraint based on the muscle tension in the limb. Also, tongue chewing was reduced by consequating it with a trainer's grasping and squeezing clients' cheeks with index finger and thumb (Aurand, Sission, Aach, & Van Hasselt, 1987), a technique some have also used to reduce grinding of teeth. Caution must be exercised in using physical restraint as a punisher, however, given that Favell, McGimsey, and Jones (1978) demonstrated that it served as a reinforcer for some people with developmental disabilities who engaged in self-injurious behaviors.

Forms of physical restraint have been used to treat behaviors other than self-injury. After having taught retarded children to walk, O'Brien, Azrin, and Bugle (1972) used short manual restraint as a consequence to reduce their crawling. Giles and Wolf (1966) used a form of restraint to decrease toileting accidents. Henricksen and Doughty (1967) and O'Brien, Bugle, and Azrin (1972) used response interruption and restraint in teaching proper mealtime skills. Koegel, Firestone, Kramme, and Dunlap (1974) used short manual restraint of the relevant body part as a consequence to reduce self-stimulation by youngsters with autism.

Whenever use is made of manual guidance, researchers are restraining limbs from performing some actions while prompting particular skills. Yet, we will devote no more attention in this section to the physical restraint inherent in the use of manual guidance.

Response Cost

Response cost is the removal of reinforcers as a consequence for a behavior (Azrin & Holz, 1966; Matson & DiLorenzo, 1984; Pazulinec, Meyerrose, & Sajwaj, 1983). Normally, we encounter this type of punishment when we delay payment of bills (late fees) and when we are fined for legal infractions (e.g., traffic tickets). Children have toys taken from them when they misuse them (e.g., bang blocks against stereos) and adults lose jobs for working under the influence of intoxicating substances. Readers should note the similarity between response cost and time-out (reinforcers are removed as a consequence in both instances), but also note the difference—there is no specified period of loss in response cost.

One type of response cost is interpreted within the concept of a chain schedule of reinforcement—a schedule in which the reinforcer occurs only after the completion of separate component behaviors (Pazulinec et al., 1983). For example, Sajwaj and Risley (1970) had a girl with mental retardation practice writing the alphabet from A to Z, after which she could listen to her favorite album. To reduce her errors, she was required to begin writing again from the letter A whenever an error occurred. In the attempt to get children with mental retardation to stop crawling mentioned earlier (O'Brien et al., 1972), whenever the children were caught crawling, they were returned to the place they had begun (response cost) and prompted to walk where they wanted to go. Cipani (1981) reduced spilling food while eating by awarding a token for three consecutive responses without spilling. Response cost occurred after a spill by cancelling the one or two correct responses that may have occurred before the spill. In teaching multiple discriminations to students with mental retardation (i.e., naming colors, numbers, and alphabet letters), O'Brien (1978) used a counter that advanced in steps, one step for each correct response. When the counter was fully advanced, the student was given a reinforcer (e.g., a bite of food or an ounce of drink). Response cost was provided by resetting the counter to the beginning immediately after an error.

Typically, however, response cost is used in treatments that provide clients with conditioned reinforcers (e.g., tokens and points) that can be later exchanged for backup reinforcers. In these treatments, response cost consists of taking the conditioned reinforcers from the clients for misbehaviors. Pazulinec et al. (1983) classified the response cost techniques into three categories: (a) the clients are given the conditioned reinforcers noncontingently, (b) the clients earn the conditioned reinforcers by performing adaptive behaviors, and (c) the clients are divided into groups and they get and lose conditioned reinforcers depending on their group's performance.

Kazdin (1973) used withdrawal of tokens to reduce speech dysfluencies (e.g., echolalia) in 40 people with mental retardation. Gregory (1972) used response cost to reduce misbehaviors of adolescents with mild mental retardation in a special education classroom. Adolescents with mild mental retardation in a state institution learned to suppress antisocial behavior when response cost was used as a consequence (Burchard & Barrera, 1972). Finally, women with severe and profound mental retardation learned to suppress self-stimulatory behaviors when these were consequated with response cost (Wrighton, 1978).

Overcorrection

Overcorrection is another type of punishment that is difficult to classify and therefore generally requires a section unto itself. It includes time-out, typically involves restraint, might involve extinction, and includes avoidance and escape (Foxx & Bechtel, 1983). Regardless, overcorrection is punishment in that it is provided as a consequence for a behavior and, when so provided, the frequency of that behavior decreases.

The overcorrection rationale is to make clients responsible for their behaviors. This is accomplished by consequating misbehaviors with a requirement to "overcorrect" the disturbance created by the misbehavior and/or to overly practice relevant correct forms of behavior (Foxx & Bechtel, 1983). The former is typically called *overcorrection/restitution;* the latter, *overcorrection/positive practice.*

In overcorrection, the trainer reprimands the client for the misbehavior immediately after it occurs, tells the client what to do as a consequence, and provides graduated guidance to get the client to do it. When providing graduated guidance, trainers typically tell clients what to do and shadow them. If clients do not respond to the instruction, trainers begin within seconds providing as little manual guidance as is needed to get them to perform as instructed. At times, clients may generate much struggle with trainers in performing as required. Because clients are relieved of the restraint inherent in manual guidance when they perform as instructed, the clients are motivated in graduated guidance by avoidance and escape. Trainers use no praise or other reinforcers during restitution or positive practice. The restitution and positive practice periods typically last from 5 to 10 minutes, although some periods have been as short as 2 minutes and others as long as 2 hours (Foxx & Bechtel, 1983).

One example of positive practice has been called "functional movement training," and is the one most often used (Foxx & Bechtel, 1983). Foxx and Azrin (1973a) used functional movement training as a consequence for self-stimulatory behavior with four youngsters with severe/profound mental retardation. To decrease a child's headweaving, the trainers reprimanded her, restrained her head, and then instructed her to move it in one of three directions (up, down, or straight ahead) and to maintain it in that position for 15 seconds. The trainer then prompted her to move it in another of the three directions and maintain it for 15 seconds, and so forth, doing so for 5 minutes following each instance of headweaving. To decrease handclapping, the trainers used 5 hand positions in the overcorrection requirement that occurred as a consequence (above the head, straight out in front, in pockets, held together, and behind the back). Azrin, Kaplan, and Foxx (1973) reduced bodyrocking by having clients maintain their shoulders away from and against the backs of chairs. To reduce flipping paper with fingers, they had the clients practice three hand positions (above the head, outstretched from the sides of the body, and against the sides of the bodies). Trainers required this practice for 20 minutes after each instance of self-stimulation, as was done with the headweaving child discussed earlier, when 5-minute periods produced inadequate reduction.

An example of restitution has been called "oral hygiene training," and was used by Foxx and Azrin (1973a) to reduce mouthing of objects by two youngsters with profound mental retardation. The potential disturbance created by mouthing objects is exposure to harmful microorganisms in the mouths of clients. Thus, when the children mouthed something, the trainers reprimanded them, had them go to the bathroom, brush their mouths with toothbrushes soaked in an antiseptic mouthwash, and wipe their lips with washcloths. Another example of restitution called "cleanliness training" is used for reducing toileting accidents. Cleanliness training typically involves getting the client to clean the mess on the floor, chair, and so on, properly dispose of the soiled clothing, clean their bodies, and dress themselves (Foxx & Azrin, 1973b).

Foxx and Bechtel (1983) described "quiet training" as using graduated guidance to keep a client from thrashing about, leaving the scene, or moving violently for 10 to 15 minutes after engaging in agitation (e.g., aggression, property destruction, or creating a commotion). The rationale was to get agitated clients to relax as a consequence for agitated behaviors. Although these authors referred to this as a *restitution* procedure (i.e., overcorrect the disturbance), it may also be considered a *positive practice* consequence (i.e., overly practice a relevant correct form of behavior).

Regardless, researchers have used overcorrection in the specific sense detailed by Foxx and Bechtel (1983) and in procedures that include many of the parameters of overcorrection in countless numbers of studies with people who have developmental disabilities. They have included reducing aggression, self-injurious behaviors, scavenging, pica, caprophagy, mealtime misbehaviors, toileting accidents, classroom disruption, self-stimulation, errors in instruction, public masturbation, stealing, floor sprawling, stripping of clothing, drooling, and other behaviors. Interested readers are referred to Foxx and Bechtel (1983) and to Matson and DiLorenzo (1984) for excellent reviews of this voluminous literature.

Contingent Electric Shock

Contingent electric shock has received more negative press than other methods of punishment and has been all but banned from use in some states (Matson & DiLorenzo, 1984). Carr and Lovaas (1983) recommended limiting consideration of its use to a very restrictive list of problems. Yet, as Repp and Deitz (1978) reminded us, serious maladaptive behaviors of clients in our charge require treatment, and when we are unable to adequately reduce these with other techniques, disregarding any proven effective treatment out of hand seems unethical, and is probably illegal.

Matson and DiLorenzo (1984) described *contingent electric shock* as the presentation of an electrical change immediately following misbehavior through two electrodes placed on the misbehaver's fingers, forearms, legs, or feet. These electrodes are attached to the clients with strips of cloth or elastic. For Carr and Lovaas (1983), the current is delivered from a handheld device (shock stick) that has two protruding electrodes at its end. The shock stick includes from 3 to 5 flashlight batteries of 1.5 volts each to provide electricity to its self-contained inductorium device. (Earlier devices required household current.) The shock sticks deliver a peak shock of 1400 volts at

0.4 milliamperes. The clients feel the shock as the electrical charge passes through their skin between the electrodes. The shock has been reported to feel like one has been hit with a willow switch or leather strap. Yet, the pain is localized, does not radiate, and stops as soon as the shock is terminated (typically within 0.5 to 2 seconds), leaving no apparent injury to the tissue (Carr & Lovaas, 1983).

Matson and DiLorenzo (1984) noted that different researchers have devised variant methods of shock administration. To allow clients greater freedom of movement, for example, some used systems with very long wires. Others developed methods of administering the shock via remote control devices. More recently, devices have been devised that deliver shock automatically when clients perform certain self-injurious behaviors. Currently, one automatic device, SIBIS (Self-Injurious Behavior Inhibiting System), has been entered into the debate regarding whether punishment is ever needed. This battery-powered shock device is headgear designed by Johns Hopkins University to reduce headbanging. SIBIS has received much press coverage emphasizing that the parents of a daughter with developmental disabilities found special educators and psychologists inept until they used SIBIS (Snell, 1987).

Researchers using shock have generally treated people with developmental disabilities (Carr & Lovaas, 1983; Matson & DiLorenzo, 1984). Most interventions involved the treatment of self-injurious behaviors, including headbanging, face slapping, and biting and/or chewing on body parts. Matson and DiLorenzo (1984) listed over 15 studies showing the suppression of self-injurious behaviors with contingent electric shock. They also listed studies of reducing tantrums, screaming, chronic ruminative vomiting, whining, aggression, property destruction, self-stimulation, and self-induced convulsions ("seizures").

In their thorough review, Carr and Lovaas (1983) summarized the various parameters that effect successful treatment with contingent electric shock. Most of these parameters are those addressed earlier that apply to all punishment (e.g., concern with developing and reinforcing alternative behaviors, immediacy, continuous rather than intermittent administration, avoiding establishment of the shock as a discriminative stimulus, and ensuring that no escape from the shock is possible). Carr and Lovaas also reviewed the noted side effects of contingent electric shock and concluded that the untoward effects others have expected (e.g., emotional responses and aggression) generally do not occur. More likely to occur are positive side effects, and they note many. Matson and DiLorenzo (1984) joined them in concluding that the positive side effects far outweigh the negative ones.

Other Types of Punishment

Both Bailey (1983) and Matson and DiLorenzo (1984) provided reviews of a number of punishers that have been used effectively but cannot be included in the categories above. Bailey separated these punishers into the following categories: aversive sounds, smells, and tastes; removal or distortion of visual stimuli; and novel aversive physical sensations. Matson and DiLorenzo generally covered these punishers under the categories of noxious substances and other forms of punishing stimuli. Little of this research will be mentioned in this chapter, and readers are encouraged to read these reviews.

Kazdin (1973) used noise at 80 decibels to consequate and thereby reduce speech dysfluencies (e.g., stammering) in people with mental retardation. Tanner and Zeiler (1975) broke ammonia capsules and held them near the face of a woman as a consequence for her slapping herself and thereby eliminating this behavior. Mayhew and Harris (1979) put lemon juice in the mouth of a man with profound mental retardation for screaming and hitting himself, substantially reducing both behaviors. Dorsey, Iwata, Ong, and McSween (1980) sprayed a fine mist of water into the faces of people with mental retardation for self-injurious behaviors and demonstrated that the water mist was an effective punisher. Similarly, Carr and Lovaas (1983) reported effective treatment using puffs of air in clients' eyes or requiring them to exercise as a consequence for a misbehavior. Other punishers mentioned in cited reviews include hair pulls, slaps to thighs with a wooden ruler, aversive tickling, cold showers, and shaving cream.

Other types of punishment are typically considered *alternatives* to punishment (cf., Matson & DiLorenzo, 1984). Differential reinforcement of other behavior (DRO), for example, can be described as reinforcement for going a period of time without performing a target misbehavior. But, as Axelrod (1987) noted, reinforcement is defined by an increase in the frequency of a behavior. Yet, studies using DRO ("omission training") record only decreases in misbehaviors. An example of DRO such as getting a token for every 3 minutes without performing self-injury could be better analyzed as punishment. In this analysis, the misbehavior results in delaying the receipt of the token reinforcement by as much as 3 minutes. The delay is a period of less reinforcement, much like time-out (Matson & DiLorenzo, 1984).

In a similar analysis, DRL (differential reinforcement of low rates) is also better understood as punishment (Axelrod, 1987). This procedure is like DRO, except that some minimum number of the misbehaviors may occur during a period of time and the client will still be given the reinforcer. For example, the client will get a token if during a 10-minute interval of time, no more than 3 face slaps have occurred. If more than 3 slaps occur during the interval, the client will not get the scheduled token reinforcement for that period. Again, the consequence of the misbehavior is less reinforcement, the results are reductions in behavior, and this is punishment.

A similar analysis can be provided for another reduction method, called *differential reinforcement of incompatible behavior* (DRI). In DRI, reinforcement is provided for behaviors that are topographically incompatible with the misbehavior. Matson and DiLorenzo (1984) discussed the time-out involved in a DRI program that used vibrating back massage as a reinforcer for appropriate use of hands to decrease a client's hitting her head. When the client was receiving massage and she hit herself, the massager was turned off (response cost).

Unfortunately, the types of analysis given to DRO, DRL, and DRI border on word games in which those opposed to punishment are more apt to call them *reinforcement*. The arguments are similar to some word games used to avoid delaying treatments until they are reviewed by some regulatory entity. Given that regulators require such review for punishing misbehaviors during meals by disallowing seconds as a consequence (response cost), one can provide the same punishment procedure by calling it reinforcement—seconds are earned by eating the meal without misbehaviors. The same procedure by another name and description avoids regulation. Unfortunately, neither space nor time allows for a thorough review of all of the techniques that are called reinforcement but that could better be analyzed as punishment or, at least, could include punishment. Suffice it to say that when the target behavior is a maladaptive one and treatment results in a decrease of that behavior, the treatment methods may best be analyzed as punishment, regardless of what the author names it.

CONCLUDING REMARKS

At the time of this writing, much controversy exists as to using punishment in treating people with disabilities (Axelrod, 1987). One organization with many professionals, The Association for Persons with Severe Handicaps, essentially rejected the use of punishment in treatment. This position was soon enjoined by the Association for Retarded Citizens. In part because of the information networks of these organizations, regulatory agencies and the federal and state governments spewed forth laws and restrictive regulations. Also, the nation was informed by the press and television of a dispute in Massachusetts regarding the use of punishment. The dispute was between a regulation agency and the parents of people with autism. Yet, demonstrations of the benefits of punishment in reducing misbehaviors of people with disabilities continue to be published, as do reviews of the punishment literature such as the present chapter.

Some are pleased with the outcome of the Massachusetts dispute mentioned above (Lindsley, 1987). As parents of a youngster with autism finally saw their son's behavior patterns improve, a regulation agency forced his treatment team to stop using punishment. Their son returned to performing his maladaptive patterns. His parents organized other parents, engaged a competent attorney, and went to court. The legal proceedings concluded with a new method of punishment regulation, *substitutive judgment*. The judges "substitute" themselves for the clients and decide whether to use the punishment on the basis of the effects of the treatment on the clients' behaviors. Lindsley noted that this evaluation method is one more like that of behavior analysts, one based on the behavioral effects of therapeutic punishment. This method contrasts with more typical regulations that base decisions on normalcy, whether all less intrusive methods have first been tried and found wanting, and whether the punishment procedure is banned by law or regulation.

Some would prefer that the regulation of punishment be limited to evaluation by a behavior analyst operating within the guidelines of the Association for Advancement of Behavior Therapy (1977). Unfortunately, the use of punishment is typically regulated by others restricting its use until it is first approved by a licensed physician or psychologist, a behavior analyst, and/or a transdisciplinary team. Some procedures might also require prior approval from a behavior management committee and others entail additional reviews by a human rights committee. Suffice it to say that any personnel considering the use of punishment would do well to know the regulations required by the status of their clients and to adhere to the relevant guidelines and regulations. Only in this manner can people with developmental disabilities obtain the benefits of therapeutic punishment (cf., Griffith, 1983; Matson & DiLorenzo, 1984).

REFERENCES

Abramowitz, A. J., & O'Leary, S. J. (1987, November). Peer mediators of the delayed reprimand effect. Poster presented at the 21st Annual Convention of the Association for Advancement of Behavior Therapy, Boston.

Alexander, F. G., & Selesnick, S. T. (1966). *The history of psychiatry: An evaluation of psychiatric thought and practice from prehistoric times to the present*. New York: Harper & Row.

Association for Advancement of Behavior Therapy. (1977). Ethical issues for human service. *Behavior Therapy, 8*, 763–764.

Augustine, A., & Cipani, E. (1982). Treating self-injurious behavior: Initial effects, maintenance and acceptability of treatment. *Child and Family Behavior Therapy, 4*(4), 53–69.

Aurand, J. C., Sisson, L. A., Aach, S. R., & Van Hasselt, V. B. (1987, November). Use of reinforcement plus interruption to reduce stereotyped self-stimulation in a blind multihandicapped child. Paper presented at the 21st Annual Convention of the Association for Advancement of Behavior Therapy, Boston.

Axelrod, S. (1987). Doing it without arrows: A review of LaVigna and Donnellan's *Alternatives to punishment: Solving behavior problems with non-aversive strategies. The Behavior Analyst, 10,* 243–251.

Axelrod, S., & Apsche, J. (Eds.). (1983). *The effects of punishment on human behavior.* New York: Academic Press.

Azrin, N. H., & Holz, W. C. (1966). Punishment. In W. K. Honig (Ed.), *Operant behavior: Areas of research and application* (pp. 380–447). New York: Appleton-Century-Crofts.

Azrin, N. H., Kaplan, S. J., & Foxx, R. M. (1973). Autism reversal: Eliminating stereotyped self-stimulation of retarded individuals. *American Journal of Mental Deficiency, 78,* 241–248.

Bailey, S. L. (1983). Extraneous aversives. In S. Axelrod and J. Apsche (Eds.), *The effects of punishment on human behavior* (pp. 247–284). New York: Academic Press.

Barrett, B. H. (1969). Behavior modification in the home: Parents adapt laboratory-developed tactics to bowel-train a 5½-year-old. *Psychotherapy: Theory, Research and Practice, 6,* 172–176.

Baumeister, A. A., & Forehand, R. (1972). Effects of contingent shock and verbal command on body rocking of retardates. *Journal of Clinical Psychology, 28,* 586–590.

Baumeister, A. A., & Rollings, J. P. (1976). Self-injurious behavior. In N. R. Ellis (Ed.), *International review of research in mental retardation.* New York: Academic Press.

Bostow, D., & Bailey, J. B. (1969). Modification of severe disruptive and aggressive behavior using brief timeout and reinforcement procedures. *Journal of Applied Behavior Analysis, 2,* 31–37.

Brantner, J. P., & Doherty, M. A. (1983). A review of timeout: A conceptual and methodological analysis. In S. Axelrod & J. Apsche (Eds.), *The effects of punishment on human behavior* (pp. 87–132). New York: Academic Press.

Bucher, B., Reykdal, B., & Albin, J. (1976). Brief physical restraint to control pica in retarded children. *Journal of Behavior Therapy and Experimental Psychiatry, 7,* 137–140.

Burchard, J. D., & Barrera, F. (1972). An analysis of timeout and response cost in a programmed environment. *Journal of Applied Behavior Analysis, 5,* 271–279.

Carlson, C. S., Arnold, C. R., Becker, W. C., & Madsen, C. H. (1968). The elimination of tantrum behavior of a child in an elementary classroom. *Behavior Research and Therapy, 6,* 117–119.

Carr, E. G., & Lovaas, I. O. (1983). Contingent shock treatment for behavior problems. In S. Axelrod & J. Apsche (Eds.), *The effects of punishment on human behavior* (pp. 221–245). New York: Academic Press.

Cipani, E. (1981). Modifying food spillage behavior in an institutionalized retarded client. *Journal of Behavior Therapy and Experimental Psychiatry, 12,* 261–265.

Cipani, E., & Wolter, J. (1983). The effectiveness of immobilization in treating self-injurious behavior. *Behavioral Engineering, 8*(4), 154–158.

Davis, J. M., & Gierl, B. (1984). Pharmacological treatment in the care of schizophrenic patients. In A. S. Bellack (Ed.) *Schizophrenia: Treatment, management, and rehabilitation* (pp. 133–173). Orlando, FL: Grune & Stratton, Inc.

Dorsey, M. F., Iwata, B. A., Ong, P., & McSween, T. E. (1980). Treatment of self-injurious behavior using a water mist: Initial response suppression and generalization. *Journal of Applied Behavior Analysis, 13,* 343–353.

Favell, J. E., McGimsey, J. F., & Jones, M. L. (1978). The use of physical restraint in the treatment of self-injury and as positive reinforcement. *Journal of Applied Behavior Analysis, 11,* 225–241.

Ferster, C. B., & Skinner, B. F. (1957). *Schedules of reinforcement.* New York: Appleton-Century-Crofts.

Foxx, R. M., & Azrin, N. H. (1973a). The elimination of autistic self-stimulatory behavior by overcorrection. *Journal of Applied Behavior Analysis, 6,* 1–14.

Foxx, R. M., & Azrin, N. H. (1973b). Dry pants: A rapid method of toilet training children. *Behavior Research and Therapy, 11,* 435–442.

Foxx, R. M., & Bechtel, D. R. (1983). Overcorrection: A review and analysis. In S. Axelrod & J. Apsche (Eds.), *The effects of punishment on human behavior* (pp. 133–220). New York: Academic Press.

Foxx, R. M., & Shapiro, S. T. (1978). The timeout ribbon: A nonexclusionary timeout procedure. *Journal of Applied Behavior Analysis, 11,* 125–136.

Franks, C. M. (1984). Foreword. In J. L. Matson & T. M. DiLorenzo, *Punishment and its alternatives: A new perspective for behavior modification* (pp. ix–xiv). New York: Springer Publishing Company.

Giles, D. K., & Wolf, M. M. (1966). Toilet training institutionalized, severe retardates: An application of operant behavior modification procedures. *American Journal of Mental Deficiency, 70,* 766–780.

Gregory, L. A. (1972). The relative effectiveness of positive reinforcement and response cost procedures in a token reinforcement program in two special education classes in a junior high school. Unpublished doctoral dissertation. Ohio State University.

Griffith, R. G. (1983). The administrative issues: An ethical and legal perspective. In S. Axelrod and J. Apsche (Eds.), *The effects of punishment on human behavior* (pp. 317–338). New York: Academic Press.

Hall, R. V., Axelrod, S., Foundopoulos, M., Shellman, J., Campbell, R. A., & Cranston, S. S. (1971). The effective use of punishment to modify behavior in the classroom. *Educational Technology, 11,* 24–26.

Hamilton, J., Stephens, K., & Allen, P. (1967). Controlling aggressive and destructive behavior in severely retarded institutionalized residents. *American Journal of Mental Deficiency, 71,* 852–856.

Harris, S. L., & Wolchik, S. A. (1979). Suppression of self-stimulation: Three alternative strategies. *Journal of Applied Behavior Analysis, 12,* 185–198.

Henricksen, K., & Doughty, R. (1967). Decelerating undesirable mealtime behavior in a group of profoundly retarded boys. *American Journal of Mental Deficiency, 72,* 40–44.

Hobbs, S. A., Forehand, R., & Murray, R. G. (1978). Effects of various durations of timeout on the noncompliant behavior of children. *Behavior Therapy, 9,* 652–656.

Johnston, J. M. (1972). Punishment of human behavior. *American Psychologist, 27,* 1033–1054.

Jones, F. J., & Miller, W. H. (1974). The effective use of negative attention for reducing group disruption in special elementary school classrooms. *Psychological Record, 24,* 435–448.

Kazdin, A. E. (1973). The effect of response cost and aversive stimulation in suppressing punished and nonpunished speech dysfluencies. *Behavior Therapy, 4,* 73–82.

Kazdin, A. E., Firestone, P. B., Kramme, K. W., & Dunlap, G. (1974). Increasing spontaneous play by suppressing self-stimulation in autistic children. *Journal of Applied Behavior Analysis, 7,* 521–528.

Lindsley, O. R. (1987). The ABA humanitarian awards for the right to effective treatment: Presentations to Robert A. Sherman and Claudia and Leo Soucy. *The Behavior Analyst, 10,* 241–242.

Lovaas, O. I., & Simmons, J. Q. (1969). Manipulations of self-destruction in three retarded children. *Journal of Applied Behavior Analysis, 2,* 143–157.

Lutzker, J. R. (1978). Reducing self-injurious behavior by facial screening. *American Journal of Mental Deficiency, 82,* 510–513.

Matson, J. L., & DiLorenzo, T. M. (1984). *Punishment and its alternatives: A new perspective for behavior modification.* New York: Springer Publishing Company, Inc.

May, J. G., Risley, T. R., Twardosz, S., Friedman, P., Bijou, S., & Wexler, D. (1975). *Guidelines for the use of behavioral procedures in state programs for retarded persons.* Arlington, TX: National Association for Retarded Citizens.

Mayhew, G., & Harris, F. (1979). Decreasing self-injurious behavior: Punishment with citric acid and reinforcement of alternative behaviors. *Behavior Modification, 3,* 322–336.

Michael, J. L. (1982). Distinguishing between discriminative and motivational functions of stimuli. *Journal of the Experimental Analysis of Behavior, 37,* 149–155.

Morse, W. H., & Kelleher, R. T. (1977). Determinants of reinforcement and punishment. In W. K. Honig & J. E. R. Staddon (Eds.), *Handbook of operant behavior.* Englewood Cliffs, NJ: Prentice-Hall.

O'Brien, F. (1978). An error-free, quick, and enjoyed strategy for teaching multiple discriminations to severely delayed students. *Mental Retardation, 16,* 291–294.

O'Brien, F. (1981). Treating self-stimulatory behavior. In J. L. Matson & J. R. McCartney (Eds.), *Handbook of behavior modification with the mentally retarded* (pp. 117–150). New York: Plenum Press.

PUNISHMENT 57

O'Brien, F., & Azrin, N. H. (1970). Behavioral engineering: Control of posture by informational feedback. *Journal of Applied Behavior Analysis, 3*, 235–240.

O'Brien, F., & Azrin, N. H. (1972). Developing proper mealtime behaviors of the institutionalized retarded. *Journal of Applied Behavior Analysis, 5*, 389–399.

O'Brien, F., Azrin, N. H., & Bugle, C. (1972). Training profoundly retarded children to stop crawling. *Journal of Applied Behavior Analysis, 5*, 131–137.

O'Brien, F., Bugle, C., & Azrin, N. H. (1972). Training and maintaining a retarded child's proper eating. *Journal of Applied Behavior Analysis, 5*, 67–72.

Pazulinec, R., Meyerrose, M., & Sajwaj, T. (1983). Punishment via response cost. In S. Axelrod & J. Apsche (Eds.), *The effects of punishment on human behavior* (pp. 71–86). New York: Academic Press.

Porterfield, J. K., Herbert-Jackson, E., & Risley, T. R. (1976). Contingent observation: An effective and acceptable procedure for reducing disruptive behavior of young children in a group setting. *Journal of Applied Behavior Analysis, 9*, 55–64.

Repp, A. C., & Brulle, A. R. (1981). Reducing aggressive behavior of mentally retarded persons. In J. L. Matson & J. R. McCartney (Eds.), *Handbook of behavior modification with the mentally retarded* (pp. 177–210). New York: Plenum Press.

Repp, A. C., & Deitz, D. E. D. (1978). On the selective use of punishment: Suggested guidelines for administrators. *Mental Retardation, 16*, 250–254.

Repp, A. C., Deitz, S. M., & Speir, N. C. (1974). Reducing stereotypic responding of retarded persons by the differential reinforcement of other behaviors. *Journal of Mental Deficiency, 79*, 279–284.

Risley, T. (1968). The effects and side effects of punishing the autistic behaviors of a deviant child. *Journal of Applied Behavior Analysis, 1*, 21–34.

Risley, T. R., & Wolf, M. M. (1967). Establishing functional speech in echolalic children. *Behaviour Research and Therapy, 5*, 73–88.

Sajwaj, T., & Risley, T. (1970). Development and generalization of writing skills in a retarded girl using manipulations of task variables. *Proceedings of the 78th Annual Convention of the American Psychological Association, 5*, 749–750.

Sajwaj, T., Culver, P., Hall, C., & Lehr, L. (1972). Three simple punishment techniques for the control of classroom disruptions. In G. Semb (Ed.), *Behavior analysis and education* (pp. 331–341). Lawrence: University of Kansas.

Schroeder, S. R., Peterson, C., Solomon, L., & Artley, J. (1977). EMG feedback and the contingent restraint of self-injurious behavior among the severely retarded: Two case illustrations. *Behavior Therapy, 8*, 738–741.

Schroeder, S. R., Schroeder, C. S., Rojahn, J., & Mulick, J. A. (1981). Self-injurious behavior: An analysis of behavior management techniques. In J. L. Matson & J. R. McCartney (Eds.), *Handbook of behavior modification with the mentally retarded* (pp. 61–115). New York: Plenum Press.

Schutz, R., Wehman, P., Renzaglia, A., & Karan, O. (1978). Efficacy of contingent social disapproval on inappropriate verbalization of two severely retarded males. *Behavior Therapy, 9*, 657–662.

Snell, M. E. (1987). In response to Axelrod's review of *Alternatives to punishment. The Behavior Analyst, 10*, 295–297.

Spencer, T., & Lutzker, J. R. (1974, August). Punishment of self-injurious behavior in retardates by application of a harmless face cover. Paper presented at the meeting of the American Psychological Association, New Orleans, LA.

Tanner, B. A., & Zeiler, M. (1975). Punishment of self-injurious behavior using aromatic ammonia as the aversive stimulus. *Journal of Applied Behavior Analysis, 8*, 53–57.

Torrey, E. F. (1983). *Surviving schizophrenia.* New York: Harper & Row.

Van Houten, R. (1983). Punishment: From the animal laboratory to the applied setting. In S. Axelrod & J. Apsche (Eds.), *The effects of punishment on human behavior* (pp. 13–44). New York: Academic Press.

Van Houten, R., & Doleys, D. M. (1983). Are social reprimands effective? In S. Axelrod & J. Apsche (Eds.), *The effects of punishment on human behavior* (pp. 45–70). New York: Academic Press.

Webster, D. R., & Azrin, N. H. (1973). Required relaxation: A method of inhibiting agitative-disruptive behavior of retardates. *Behavior Research and Therapy, 11,* 67–78.

Webster's ninth new collegiate dictionary. (1987). Springfield, MA: Merriam-Webster, Inc.

Wolf, M. M., Risley, T. R., & Mees, H. L. (1964). Application of operant conditioning procedures to the behavior problems of an autistic child. *Behaviour Research and Therapy, 1,* 305–312.

Wolfensberger, W. (1972). *The principle of normalization in human services.* Toronto: National Institute on Mental Retardation.

Wrighton, P. (1978). Comparative effects of demerit tokens, response cost, and time out to decrease self-stimulatory behavior during posture training with severely and profoundly retarded women. Unpublished doctoral dissertation, University of Manitoba.

Zegiob, L. E., Jenkins, J., Becker, J., & Bristow, A. (1976). Facial screening: Effects on appropriate and inappropriate behaviors. *Journal of Behavior Therapy and Experimental Psychiatry, 7,* 355–357.

The Role of Positive Programming in Behavioral Treatment

Gary W. LaVigna
and
Thomas J. Willis
Institute for Applied Behavior Analysis,
Los Angeles

Anne M. Donnellan
University of Wisconsin, Madison

This chapter defines and describes the role of positive programming in the treatment of the severe behavior problems often exhibited by individuals who face the challenge of a severely handicapping condition. After discussing the context and need for positive programming within a conceptual framework for research and treatment based on outcome needs, variations within this strategy are delineated. Then, assessment and analysis are described as critical for comprehensive, positive, and effective treatment. A case study of severe aggression is then presented in detail to illustrate the process of assessment and analysis, the treatment program that follows from this process, and the long term results of this approach to intervention. Finally, conclusions are drawn that examine the implications of positive programming for the future role of aversive procedures in the behavioral treatment of children, adolescents, and adults and for the practice of applied behavior analysis in the field of developmental disabilities.

DEFINITION

Although the term *positive programming* can refer to the universe of nonaversive strategies, in this chapter it has a more specific meaning (Donnellan, LaVigna, Negri-Shoultz, & Fassbender, 1988; LaVigna & Donnellan, 1986). *Positive programming* is defined as a longitudinal, instructional program designed to give the learner greater skills and competencies for the

Acknowledgment. The authors wish to thank Don Fender, Joanne Duncan, Pat McCarthy, and the staff of the treatment home in Lexington, Kentucky, for their cooperation in the case study reported in this chapter.

purpose of controlling or eliminating problem behavior in order to facilitate and enhance social integration. Positive programming, in this sense, is based on a functional analysis of the presenting problem and involves the systematic manipulation of stimulus conditions, consequences, instructional stimuli, and other variables in an effort to establish the new, more adaptive behavioral repertoire.

THE CONTEXT AND NEED
FOR POSITIVE PROGRAMMING

While punitive procedures may produce rapid and sharp suppression of problematic behaviors, serious questions about the durability and generalization of treatment effects, side effects, and social validity suggest that the present punishment technology has narrow utility and is of little if any value for true community and social integration (LaVigna, 1987). For example, in an exemplary follow-up study of the original overcorrection reports, the findings were quite remarkable (Foxx & Livesay, 1984). Four of the original cases involved pica behavior. On follow-up 10 years later, three of the four had died, although the causes of death were not determined. While this is an unusual and extreme finding, generally, for all cases, the effects of treatment disappeared as the researcher left the setting. Foxx and Livesay concluded that the field should become less concerned with speed and degree of effects and become more concerned with duration of effects.

As suggested above, procedural efficacy is measured by a variety of outcome criteria. In addition to the traditional speed and degree of effects, these criteria also include the durability and generalization of effects and side effects, and the social validity of the procedures being implemented (Association for the Advancement of Behavior Therapy, 1982). This array of critical treatment outcomes makes it unlikely that any one procedure will produce all of the desired results. Rather, full results are likely to require multielement treatment plans the various components of which, in combination, address the full range of outcome requirements.

THE DESIGN OF
TREATMENT PROGRAMS

The integration of these separate components into an organized treatment plan is illustrated in Figure 1. The first major distinction is between *reactive strategies* and *proactive strategies*. The main goal of a reactive strategy is to establish rapid control over a concrete situation to prevent injury or damage (Willis & LaVigna, 1983). Examples of reactive strategies include

PROACTIVE STRATEGIES			REACTIVE STRATEGIES
Ecological Manipulation	**Positive Programming**	**Direct Treatment**	
• Settings	• General Skills	*Behavioral*	• Active Listening
• Interactions	• Development	• Differential Schedules of Reinforcement	• Stimulus Change
• Instructional Methods	• Functional equivalent	• Stimulus Control	• Crisis Intervention
• Instructional Goals	• Functional related	• Instructional Control	
• Environmental Pollutants (e.g., noise, crowding)	• Coping/ Tolerance	• Stimulus Satiation	
• Number and Characteristics of other people		• Etc.	
		Other	
		• Neurophysical Techniques	
		• Medication Adjustments	
		• Dietary Changes	
		• Etc.	

FIGURE 1:   Organizational model for treatment planning.

stimulus change (defined as a novel and sudden but nonaversive change in ambient stimuli, producing immediate although transitory suppression in responding) (Azrin, 1958); active listening (defined as responding to the precursors or early elements in an escalating behavior problem in such a way as to remove the need for the person to continue the episode) (Gordon, 1970); and physical management procedures (Palotai, Mance, & Negri, 1982; Zivolich & Thvedt, 1983). Physical management procedures are used as a last resort.

Reactive Strategies

There are two risks in responding reactively. The first is that reactive strategy may unavoidably reinforce the target response and may therefore produce a countertherapeutic effect. Conversely, reactive strategy may contain an unavoidable aversive quality. The major danger here is that the very strategy being used to control the situation may actually contribute to its escalation through the well-documented phenomenon of punishment elicited aggression. A major goal of research should be to develop reactive strategies that minimize the potential of either reinforcing (counter-therapeutic) or aversive qualities.

Proactive Strategies

In contrast to the immediate goal of a reactive strategy, proactive strategies are those designed to decrease the frequency and/or intensity of the problematic behavior over time. Included within this category are direct treatment procedures, ecological manipulation, and, most crucially, positive programming.

Ecological Manipulation

Behaviors occur within a context and often are a function of the person's physical and interpersonal environment. *Ecological manipulation* involves planned environmental changes that in turn produce a change in behavior. As illustrated in Figure 1, examples of ecological manipulations include changing the person's setting (Horner, 1980); changing the number and quality of interactions (Egel, Richman, & Koegel, 1981; Strain, 1983); changing the instructional methods being used (Koegel, Dunlap, & Dyer, 1980; Winterling & Dunlap, 1987); changing instructional goals (Donnellan, 1980); and/or removing or controlling environmental pollutants such as noise or crowding (Adams, Tallon, & Stangl, 1980; Rago, Parker, & Cleland, 1978). Ecological manipulations attempt to "smooth the fit" between the learner and his environment by modifying the environment (Rhodes, 1967). The effectiveness of such manipulations rests on the quality of information obtained during the assessment process. Ecological manipulations can contribute significantly to the durability of treatment effects; that is, durable changes in the ecology can produce durable changes in behavior.

Direct Treatment Strategies

Ecological manipulations, depending on their complexity and/or difficulty, may take time to arrange, and positive programming may require some time before new skills and competencies are mastered. Although these strategies are likely to be necessary to produce long term treatment effects, it may also be necessary to include behavioral or other *direct treatment strategies* for more rapid effects; hence the inclusion of these strategies in treatment.

Direct Behavioral Treatment Strategies. The *direct behavioral treatment strategies* comprise a powerful but underutilized technology (LaVigna &

Donnellan, 1986). For example, two schedules of reinforcement have proved particularly useful in rapidly removing behavioral barriers to social integration: Differential Reinforcement of Other Behavior (DRO) and Differential Reinforcement of Low Rates of Responding (DRL). Although Differential Reinforcement of Incompatible Responses (DRI) and Differential Reinforcement of Alternative Responses (Alt-R) schedules are more widely used, they produce less consistent results for a variety of complex reasons (LaVigna & Donnellan, 1986; Sulzer-Azaroff & Mayer, 1977).

Within the operant paradigm, there are procedures in addition to differential schedules of reinforcement that can produce a rapid direct treatment effect (LaVigna & Donnellan, 1986). As illustrated in Figure 1, these include, but are not limited to, stimulus control (i.e., removing those stimuli that are discriminative for the problem behavior) (Touchette, 1983; Touchette, MacDonald, & Langer, 1985); instructional control (i.e., tapping rule governed behavior to establish rapid control over a problem) (Russo, Cataldo, & Cushing, 1981; Schlinger & Blakely, 1987); and stimulus satiation (i.e., reducing a behavior problem by increasing the noncontingent availability of the maintaining reinforcers) (Ayllon, 1963).

Other Direct Treatment Strategies. There are, of course, treatment strategies other than the behavioral that could play an important direct treatment role in a comprehensive intervention plan. These could include, for example, neurophysiological techniques, medication adjustments, and dietary changes (Davidson, Kleene, Carroll, & Rockowitz, 1983; Lozoff & Brittenham, 1986; Mizuno & Yugari, 1974). Direct treatment, accordingly, uses basic operant and nonoperant techniques to establish rapid control while the more permanent effects of ecological manipulations and positive programming are pursued.

Positive Programming

Ecological manipulations change the physical and interpersonal environments in which the person must interact in an effort to change those conditions associated with the problem behavior. *Positive programming* teaches more effective and socially acceptable ways of getting one's needs met and of coping with the realities of the physical and interpersonal environments in which the person must act and interact. If ecological manipulations can be described as changes in the environmental context to "smooth the fit" between the environment and the individual, positive programming can be described as changes in the person's repertoire to deal better with the environment. It is to a detailed discussion of positive programming that we now turn.

VARIATIONS OF
POSITIVE PROGRAMMING

There are four variations of positive programming. The first variation is *general skill development*, which teaches general skills in the areas of domestic, vocational, and community functioning. Two further variations of positive programming involve *specific skill development*. The first of these teaches specific skills that are *functionally equivalent* to the target behavior and the second teaches skills that are *functionally related* but not *equivalent* to the target behavior. The final variation of positive programming teaches *coping skills*, that is, effective ways of tolerating the stresses of everyday life.

Teaching General Skills

While general skills development would have value as a component of any habilitation program, it serves specific roles in a positive program to reduce problem behavior. In the first place, it is neither desirable nor possible to create nonbehaving people. This factor is of critical importance when we are working with individuals who have major skill deficits. When we eliminate a problem behavior with such people, we may create a behavioral vacuum. If the person does not have the repertoire to fill that void with a productive, socially acceptable alternative, a dynamic is created that will act against efforts toward the reduction of the problem and/or make it likely that other problems will develop. If we wish our behavior reduction efforts to have long term success, treatment efforts require that the person have the opportunity both to learn and to engage in a wide variety of meaningful tasks and activities.

The reality is that many people who are severely handicapped are in settings where they have the opportunity neither to learn nor to engage in such adaptive behaviors. These environments are often barren or at best contrived and artificial. They are absent of those contingencies that make up the fabric of challenge and reward found in the real world of natural, socially integrated settings. What often passes for programming are staff-arranged opportunities to learn and/or engage in such inappropriate and nonfunctional activities as color or shape sorting, putting pegs in boards, simulated work activities, and other repetitive, nonmeaningful tasks. This "touch-red" curriculum is so removed from the needs, interests, and potential of the person that it itself often produces problem behavior as the person's best expression of boredom, protest, frustration, anger, and the like. In contrast, a positive program, with instructional objectives that are functional and that give the person ample opportunity to learn and engage in a wide variety of relevant and/or interesting activities, would remove the conditions that are discriminative for many problem behaviors.

Chronological Age Appropriateness

There are a number of attributes that should characterize positive programming for general skill development. Tasks and materials should be chronologically age appropriate and functional and instruction should be designed to produce generalization. The suggestion that tasks and materials be *chronologically* age appropriate means that in some cases we may have to adapt a task to be *developmentally* age appropriate (Donnellan, Kosovac, & Clark, in press; Mirenda & Donnellan, 1987). For example, if we are working with an adult learner who has not yet reached the Piagetian stage of object permanence (Piaget & Inhelder, 1969), it may be necessary to have all of the ingredients for a sandwich visible in a positive program teaching independent lunch preparation. Of course, the issue of age appropriateness increases with the disparity between chronological and developmental age. The importance of this issue is twofold: the chronological age appropriateness of tasks and materials increases both the learner's dignity and our expectations of the learner. The direct and indirect effects of both of these results are very supportive of behavior change efforts. Perhaps nowhere is this impact more dramatically evident than for those of us who have had the opportunity to see the change in a person who moves from the childlike tasks of a day activity center to the adult requirements of a supported worksite in a real business setting. This has been our experience at the Institute for Applied Behavior Analysis, where we have placed over 100 adults with handicapping conditions in unsheltered, competitive jobs.

Functionality

Functionality, as a desired attribute of positive programming, has two meanings. The first is that the activity must serve a legitimate purpose (Brown, Nietupski, & Homre-Nietupski, 1976). Brown has suggested an informal but revealing way to evaluate this aspect of an activity. He suggested asking: "If the person doesn't learn to do this, will someone else have to do it for him?" For example, in many developmentally sequenced but functionally irrelevant curricula in which the individual is supposed to "point to a circle," "sort spoons from socks," or "match red felt squares and yellow felt apples," the answer would be "No." If the person did not learn such tasks, no one would have to complete the tasks for him. In asking this question about clearing the table of dirty dishes after dinner, putting the right change in the vending machine for a soda, or pointing to a picture or word card to order a hamburger at a restaurant, the answer would be "Yes!"

The second meaning of functionality in positive programming is that the activity must provide some reinforcing feedback or payoff for the person. Ideally, this payoff should be intrinsic to the task itself; if not, extrinsic reinforcement must be programmed. The implications for behavior control of a rich schedule of instruction and the opportunity to engage in activities that are both meaningful and reinforcing seem obvious. Yet rarely are such conditions available for the person exhibiting a severe behavior problem. Rather, there is an unfortunate and pervasive logic that says that behavior must be controlled before this kind of programming can begin. The suggestion here is that positive programming with the attribute of functionality is a critical strategy for behavior control itself and a necessary component of a comprehensive treatment plan.

Generalization

Finally, in addition to chronological age appropriateness and functionality, positive programming for general skill development should use low or zero inference strategies of training. Traditional training is based on a high inference model. That is, we infer that what a person learns in one setting will generalize to other settings, what a person learns on one set of materials will generalize to another set of materials, what a person learns in contrived, simulated situations and segregated settings will generalize to real situations in natural, community integrated settings. However, the more handicapped a person is, the less likely this generalization is to occur (Stokes & Baer, 1977). To avoid this problem, Donnellan and Mirenda (1983) suggested that training should occur with those tasks and materials with which and in those settings in which we want the person ultimately to perform. The same rationale applies to the control of behavior problems. Programming and intervention must take place in those settings in which we ultimately want the behavior to be under control.

To summarize, general skill development provides a general context of positive programming within which to carry out more directed efforts of behavior modification. It both increases the person's productive and socially acceptable skills and competencies *and* removes many of the conditions that are discriminative for problem behavior. Positive programming for general skill development characteristically employs tasks and materials that are chronologically age appropriate (recognizing that adaptations may be necessary to accommodate the person's developmental needs) and provides training in those settings in which the person must ultimately function.

Teaching Alternative, Functionally Equivalent Skills

A second variation of positive programming involves instruction and training to teach a *specific skill* that serves the same function as the problem behavior. A major example of this follows from the increasing characterization of aberrant behavior as a form of communication (Carr & Durand, 1985; Donnellan, Mirenda, Mesaros, & Fassbender, 1984). Positive programming in this mode attempts to identify the communicative function of the problem behavior and then to replace that behavior with an equally effective but more socially acceptable one.

Communication Training

The following are examples of this approach:

1. A person with profound mental impairments and multiple medical and physical problems would often engage in crying tantrums when alone in her bedroom. Analysis suggested that her tantrums served the function of calling staff into the room (to see what was wrong). A positive program was established to teach her to ring a bedside bell when she wanted somebody to come in (for any reason). She learned this method of calling staff and her tantrums stopped.

2. A 14-year-old teenager with the problem of autism and with no communicative speech would hit his teacher an average of six times during a 6-hour day. Typically, this would occur during a sit-down table activity. This behavior seemed to serve the communicative function of asking for a break from what he perceived as a boring activity. As an alternative, he was taught to present the teacher with a word card that said "May I have a 5-minute break please?" whenever he wanted to stop what he was doing. He was given 12 cards a day (six more opportunities for taking a break than what he was asking for during baseline conditions). He eventually used this new system of communication and stopped hitting the teacher, all for the cost of an average 10 minutes breaktime for every 50 minutes of work.

3. A 12-year-old student with a severe mental impairment but with some speech would become violently aggressive in school. This would occur 13 or more times a day. He was in a very positive and constructive environment; nevertheless, staff misunderstood how much he understood. Analysis suggested that his aggression might have been his way of expressing confusion when he did not understand what was being asked of him. First, in controlled instructional sessions he was taught to say "I'm confused, I don't understand" when the teacher made a nonsense request to him such as "gobbledeegock" or "scrooge the nod." Such requests were interspersed in a ratio of 1:3 with easily understandable requests such as "Would you get the pencil?" or "Pour the juice." Prompting and prompt fading ((Donnellan et al., 1988) were used until he consistently responded without prompting to the nonsense requests with the prescribed statement. At this point of the positive program, he

was told to be alert because he would be asked to do something he did not understand at various points throughout the schoolday. Ten randomly distributed nonsense requests were made each day and again prompt fading was used to assure his correct responding in the natural setting. As prompting was faded, he began to say "I'm confused, I don't understand" not only in response to the planned nonsense requests but also at various other times when school staff thought that they had made a perfectly reasonable and understandable request. However, each time they responded to his statements of confusion with clarification and/or simplification. He is no longer aggressive in the classroom.

In similar ways, an adolescent in a small group home was taught to say "No thank you, I would rather not" when asked to do something he did not want to do, instead of throwing a tantrum and throwing things, and a student was taught to hold up his hand when he needed help, rather than become self-injurious. In all of these examples, the communicative function of the problem behavior was identified and an alternative, more acceptable form was taught.

A major strategy for teaching an alternative form of communication to serve the function of a behavior problem is to use a communication system that will be easy and quick for the person to learn. This means taking into account the cognitive, sensory, and motor functioning of the person and the specific demands made by the different systems for discriminating and responding. There is increased awareness that traditional speech and even sign language have characteristics that make them less feasible choices in many cases, at least initially. Fortunately, the development of alternative and augmentative communication systems is becoming a field in its own right and an increasingly wide range of options is available. These options range from basic object word card and picture systems to sophisticated computerized systems.

Instructional strategies may also vary with the person or the situation. For example, if precursors to a problem behavior can be identified, their appearance may represent a *teachable moment*, an opportunity to introduce the new system and prompt its correct use. This strategy could take advantage of the naturally occurring, subsequent reinforcement to strengthen the new communication response. Or, the precursor behavior itself may represent a more desirable response that could be shaped even further by quickly responding to and reinforcing it *before* it escalates to the defined problem level.

Yet another strategy could take advantage of the routine response chains that become automatic for so many people. For example, if a person could be taught to routinely present a word card that said "I'm finished!"

prior to transitioning from any activity to another, she could begin to use that card to indicate that she had had enough of a particular task, rather than to tantrum or exhibit some other more problematic response. Or, as described above in the example of the classroom student who became aggressive when he was confused, it may be feasible to use discrete trial prompt-fading procedures to establish the alternative communication response. These or other instructional strategies can be used to teach specifically defined messages that serve a function equivalent to the one served by the problem behavior. They may utilize a communication system that is dedicated to this purpose or one that serves a broader role of communication for the person.

Independence Training

Teaching other forms of communication is not the only strategy for replacing a problem behavior with a functionally equivalent alternative. Implicit in the communication approach is reliance on another person. That is, to the extent that a problem behavior serves a communication role, it is maintained by the effectiveness with which it gets other people to respond to the expressed needs. We may reduce the problem behavior to the extent that we can teach a person to satisfy his or her own needs *independently.* The ability to perform such functionally equivalent responses would reduce the motivation for problem behavior.

An example of this is provided by one case involving a 6-year-old boy living in a small group home. He had severe intellectual impairment and exhibited high rate pica behavior (i.e., he ate inedible items, to the point that it seriously endangered his health and general well being). Among other things, a comprehensive assessment and functional analysis determined that he was not able to discriminate between edible and inedible objects and that his pica behavior was maintained by the increased opportunity to ingest. A communication strategy in this case would have inferred that his pica behavior was equivalent to his saying "I want something to eat" or "I'm hungry," and might have taught him some better way to say this. For example, pointing to a picture of various food items would allow staff to feed him something nutritious. Based on the analysis, however, the decision was made to design a positive program to increase his independence in this area.

There were two major thrusts to the positive program. The first was to teach him to discriminate between edible and inedible objects. This was accomplished through the use of a two-way forced choice, discrete trial format in which he was presented with a pebble, pencil, cotton ball, button, and so forth, paired with an almond, pretzel, marshmallow, M&M, and so forth. Ten trials per day were scheduled. If he selected the edible object, he was allowed to eat it; if he selected the inedible object, the trial was discontinued. Although learning was very gradual, he eventually would select the edible item exclusively, even when presented with items that were not used in training. He was also observed to pick an inedible object off the floor (e.g., a dust ball), look at it closely and put it down again.

The second thrust of this positive program was to teach him to prepare his own snack *anytime he wanted one*. A special floor-level cabinet in the kitchen was kept stocked with fresh fruit, dried fruit, peanuts, and other healthy items. He was the only one to receive training on how to open the latch. He eventually learned to go to his cabinet whenever he wanted to eat something. Once he learned this and could discriminate between edible and inedible items, there was no longer any reason for him to engage in pica behavior and it dropped out of his repertoire. After 4 years, the pica behavior has still not returned. (Incidentally, this youngster did not have, nor has he developed, a weight problem. He has a hollow leg.)

Teaching Alternative, Functionally Related Skills

Teaching someone to fix a sandwich when hungry, to leave a noisy, chaotic area when upset, or to put on a jacket when cold are additional examples of positive programming to teach functionally equivalent replacement behaviors for problemmatic behaviors that may have previously represented the person's best strategy for dealing with these situations. Positive programming can also develop alternative, functionally related although not directly equivalent skills. Examples of this approach include teaching choice making, schedule building, the introduction of contingency specifying stimuli, and establishing stimulus control.

We often, whether by design or accident, establish environments for our clients that are totally under staff control. We decide who will do what, where, and when. The lack of self-determined options may contribute to many behavior problems to an extent that we are only now beginning to appreciate. One justification for staff-directed activities is that many people who have severe or profound handicaps have not learned to make choices, nor do they typically have the breadth of experience that would allow them to make informed choices. In such cases, however, positive programming can be directed toward *teaching choice making behavior* and, as this skill is established, giving the person more and more control over his or her day-to-day existence.

In cases of profound intellectual impairment, this would begin at a very concrete level, using a two-way, forced choice format (as described earlier) to select from among a presented pair of items, with one clearly having reinforcement value and the other, neutral value. One choice might involve a selection between a gum drop and a copy of Shakespeare's sonnets. As a person's choice making abilities increase, choice making opportunities may be presented at increasingly abstract levels. One example of a choice making hierarchy might begin at the concrete object level, move up to pictures representing objects, then to objects representing activities, and finally to pictures representing activities.

Once a person can choose an activity by selecting an object or a picture, she can also participate in *scheduling* her own day. Organizing a day around a concrete schedule (represented by objects or pictures) is, in its own right, a positive programming strategy to reduce behavior problems. If choosing an activity provides control, the ability to use a concrete schedule provides predictability. For example, the afternoon schedule might be conveyed by a sequence of pictures or objects. The person can be oriented to the schedule and shown what activities are planned. He or she might also be reoriented to the schedule at each point of transition, with staff indicating what activity has just been finished, what is about to start, and what will follow. In addition to the person being given choices to insert at different points of the sequence, the person may also be taught to follow such a schedule independently or it can be integrated with teaching choice making.

Another strategy for establishing alternative behavior related to the identified problem involves the introduction of *contingency specifying stimuli* (Schlinger & Blakely, 1987). Some behaviors occur not because they are learned or conditioned but rather because they are under the control of some rule or statement of contingencies. Establishing new rule-governed behavior may rapidly produce new patterns of responding. For example, an adolescent boy with autism was essentially fully integrated into a regular school program and was generally doing quite well. His one remaining significant problem was his hoarding of inappropriate items in his school locker. This problem was resistant to solution until staff took advantage of the fact that he considered the student handbook his "bible." They simply typed in a new student rule: "Students are not allowed to hoard things in their lockers." The problem disappeared.

Yet another example involved an adult who had severe intellectual impairment. In his case, it was necessary to communicate the rule through a picture series. The problem behavior involved hitting his mother when she asked him to return something to the shelves in the supermarket. In fact, to avoid being hit she would let him pile up the food cart and they would end up with a bill of over $300 whenever they went shopping together. Although the intervention program for this person had many components, it included imagery-based role play practice (Groden & Cautela, 1984) to communicate to him the rule we wanted him to follow. Five times a day he was told a story about his trip to the store. The story was accompanied by a sequential series of pictures that portrayed his being in the store with his mother; his taking something off the shelf; his mother asking and pointing for him to put it back; his taking a deep breath and holding it for a count of three; his slowly releasing his breath and putting the item back as requested; and he and his mother sharing a pizza at his favorite restaurant. Other problematic situations were dealt with in a similar way. This positive programming strategy contributed to his learning new rules for behaving.

A final example of this form of positive programming involves bringing the behavior under the control of a new set of stimulus conditions. In one case, the problem behavior of a young boy involved his spitting and smearing his saliva over virtually any shiny surface, including furniture, cars, and windows. Rather than trying to eliminate this response, he was taught to engage in it only with a specially specified hand mirror. Initially, these opportunities were given to him frequently. He received differential reinforcement for engaging in this behavior under these conditions. At other times, he was simply reminded to wait for the mirror. Eventually, he learned to spit and smear his saliva only when he was given access to his mirror. At this point, staff were able to control when and where it happened. This was considered sufficient. One would not establish stimulus control over dangerous behaviors such as aggression or self-injury using this strategy, but it certainly holds promise for inappropriate verbal or other undesired but nondangerous behaviors (LaVigna & Donnellan, 1986).

Teaching Coping and Tolerance

Thus far, three varieties of positive programming have been described. The first has the aim of increasing the person's general skills and competencies across all domains; the second teaches alternative behaviors (either communicative or otherwise) that are functionally equivalent to the problem behavior; the third teaches alternative behaviors that, while not equivalent, are functionally related to the behavior we wish to decrease or eliminate. All three variations establish new behavioral repertoires that empower the individual either to influence the environment more competently or to get his or her needs met in a more socially acceptable manner. The fourth and final variation of positive programming to be discussed here teaches the person to cope with and tolerate an environment that cannot be changed and/or one in which, at least for a time, his or her needs cannot be met.

Three strategies exemplify this positive programming approach to teaching tolerance for the unavoidable stressors and naturally occurring aversive events in one's life. The first involves teaching a generalized relaxation response. Cautela and Groden (1978) have developed a particularly useful guide for teaching people with developmental disabilities how to relax when they are feeling stressed or upset. At the Groden Center, relaxation training is a standard part of the curriculum and is taught as a self-control strategy. It is not unusual to see a student guiding himself through a relaxation exercise in order to calm down when he or she is becoming tense or agitated. This self-control, stress management behavior replaces the previous repertoire of tantrums, aggression, or other undesired responding.

Another strategy for teaching tolerance is to desensitize a person to those stimulus conditions that have been associated with the problem behavior (Wolpe, 1973). For example, in one case an adult who had a severely handicapping condition would often exhibit tantrum aggression whenever in close proximity to loud noises such as another person's screaming, vacuum cleaners, floor polishers, automatic dishwashers, and so forth. The initial target was to desensitize her to screaming. A cassette tape recording was made of one of her housemate's screaming tantrums (a problem that was also being addressed). During the initial sessions, she was first guided to a state of calm and relaxation. Once this state had been achieved, the tape recorder was turned on, but at extremely low volume. To further assure that she remained calm, she was given some of her favorite food to eat. Over subsequent sessions, the volume of the tape was very gradually turned up until she could tolerate it at full volume and still stay calm and relaxed.

At this point, a similar strategy was followed to desensitize her to the vacuum cleaner. For example, in the initial session, once she was calm and relaxed the vacuum cleaner was turned on in the next room with the intervening door closed. Over subsequent sessions, the door was very gradually opened and the vacuum cleaner was moved closer and closer until she could tolerate it when it was right next to her and still stay calm and relaxed. At this point, the effects of treatment spontaneously generalized and noise no longer elicited problem behavior.

Desensitization can be programmed for criticism, crowds, or any other stimuli functionally related to the problem behavior. Another example of this variation of positive programming involves delay in reinforcement, which often is discriminative for problem behavior. How can we teach a person to be tolerant of waiting for something? In the case study presented later in this chapter, just that was taught to a young adult who previously was aggressive at least some of the time when he had to wait. Teaching him to tolerate delays contributed significantly to the treatment of his aggressive behavior.

Variations on a Theme

To summarize this section on the variations of positive programming, each variation will be illustrated as it might be applied to the same problem. For the purposes of this summary example, let us assume that the client is an adolescent who has severe handicaps and who tantrums when he is hungry. While there would very likely be other components to his treatment program, the different variations of positive programming might be as follows:

1. He could have a rich schedule of competing activities. For example, he could be taught to participate in organized recreational activities or to perform an afterschool job to help him bridge the gap from school to dinnertime.
2. He could be taught to ask for a snack when he is hungry.
3. He could be taught to fix a snack for himself when he is hungry.
4. He could be taught to schedule two to three snacks a day on his daily schedule and/or he could be oriented from time to time as to when snacks and meals will occur.
5. He could be taught to turn on the radio and listen to music to help him relax and pass the time when he has to wait for a meal.
6. Any or all of the above could be pursued simultaneously.

ASSESSMENT

The design of positive programs as described above obviously requires the most thorough and comprehensive assessment process and analysis of the presenting problem. The role of positive programming in behavioral intervention is to produce durable treatment effects. For this to occur, it is necessary to know the conditions under which the behavior occurs, the operant role it serves the person, the person's current relevant behavioral repertoire, the strengths and weaknesses of the mediating system available to implement treatment, and many other things. The fundamental role of assessment and functional analysis in behavioral intervention has strong roots in the field of applied behavior analysis (Kanfer & Saslow, 1969; Schwartz, Goldiamond, & Howe, 1975). The chapter on Behavioral Diagnostics in this volume illustrates the renewed appreciation for the role that assessment and analysis can play in the design of treatment programs.

At the Institute for Applied Behavior Analysis, we have developed a records abstraction form and information gathering instrument that serves as a comprehensive guide to the assessment process (Willis, LaVigna & Donnellan, 1987). An outline of the topics covered in this guide is presented in Table 1. Once this information is gathered, it is summarized in an assessment report following a preset format (LaVigna & Donnellan, 1986). The full application of this process is, admittedly, time consuming. However, it is justified when problems have not been solved with procedures based on less thorough information, when the problems seriously interfere with the quality of the person's life and his or her community access, and/or

TABLE 1

OUTLINE OF ASSESSMENT CONTENT

A. Referral Information.
1. General information.
2. Referral problems.
3. Treatment priority.
4. Client's or careprovider's reasons for referral.
5. Referral discrepancies.

B. Background Information.
1. Client characteristics.
   a. Physical description.
   b. Cognitive abilities.
   c. Communicative abilities.
   d. Motor/perceptual abilities.
   e. Self-care skills.
   f. Social skills.
   g. Community skills.
   h. Domestic skills.
   i. Leisure/recreation skills.
2. Family history and background.
3. Living arrangements and placement history.
4. Program placement.
5. Health and medical status.
6. Previous and current treatment.

C. Functional Analysis of Behavior.
1. Specification and measurement of the target behavior:
   a. Topography or physical description.
   b. Cycle or criteria for the beginning and ending of a response.
   c. Course or typical sequence of an episode (including possible precursors which may or may not be scored in and of themselves as a response).
   d. Strength, rate, duration, or other measures of intensity.
2. History of the problem.
   a. First appearance.
   b. Course over time.
   c. Recent increases and decreases.
   d. Cycles and other patterns.
   e. Major contributing factors.
   f. Significant contributing factors.
   g. Family factors.
   h. Medical factors.
3. Antecedent analysis:
   a. Occurrence:
      1) Settings.

TABLE 1 *Continued*

---

      2) Situations.
      3) Places.
      4) People.
      5) Time of day, week, month, and year.
      6) Immediate preceding activities, events, and interactions.
      7) Exacerbating events.
   b. Non-occurrence or absence:
      1) Settings.
      2) Situations.
      3) Places.
      4) People.
      5) Time of day, week, month, or year.
      6) Immediate preceding activities, events, and interactions.
      7) Ameliorating events.
  4. Consequence analysis:
   a. History of management methods.
   b. Current management methods.
   c. Effects of management methods.
   d. Effects of behavior on others.
   e. Effects on the environment.
   f. Reactions that exacerbate or ameliorate situation.
  5. Analysis of meaning:
   a. Hypothesis regarding functions of the behavior, e.g., communication, escape, or coercion.
   b. Hypothesis regarding maintaining payoffs or events.
   c. Hypothesis regarding what events may be suppressing alternative, more acceptable behavior.
   d. Hypothesis regarding stimuli and events discriminative for the behavior.

D. Mediator Analysis.
  1. Identify mediators.
  2. Motivation.
  3. Cooperation.
  4. Views of the problem.
  5. Emotional, physical, and technical abilities to carry out programming.
  6. Staffing resources.
  7. Factors adding to and detracting from ability to carry out programs.
  8. Estimate of resources to carry out programs.

E. Motivational Analysis.
  1. Predictable occurring behaviors.
  2. Likes and dislikes.
  3. Verbal requests.

4. Survey of preferences for:
   a. Food and beverage items.
   b. Toys and playthings (as age-appropriate).
   c. Entertainment.
   d. Sports and games.
   e. Music, arts, and crafts.
   f. Excursions and community events.
   g. Social events and interactions with others.
   h. Academic and classroom activity.
   i. Domestic activities.
   j. Work activities.
   k. Personal appearance, etc.

---

before aversive intervention is considered. However, even in cases that are being approached less formally, we would recommend that an effort be made to identify the communicative functions of the aberrant behavior. Donnellan et al. (1984) have developed a particularly useful and easy tool to use for this purpose.

CASE STUDY

The following case study illustrates the development and implementation of a comprehensive treatment program based on a thorough assessment and functional analysis and the role that positive programming plays in such an approach.

Subject

This case involved an 18-year-old young man who had the problems of autism and moderate mental retardation. He had also been previously labeled as emotionally disturbed and socially retarded. He was 6 feet tall and weighed 185 pounds. His communication system consisted primarily of gestures and short phrases, although he was difficult to understand even when he used the short phrases. He was independent in self-care. He had a variety of stereotypic behaviors, such as arm flapping, jumping, and patting himself on the chest, which he engaged in at high rates.

Setting

The setting he resided in and within which we worked was a small group home with a staff to client ratio of 1:2, which is typical in many group homes working with adults with autism who exhibit severe behavior problems (LaVigna, 1983). There also were five other adult male residents. The setting provided community-based programming, sophisticated instructional procedures, and strictly nonaversive behavior management.

Target Behavior

The behavior problem was defined as hitting, kicking, or biting another person or throwing an object in their direction. Hitting typically involved striking the other person with a downward, whole-arm movement, possibly with an object such as a broom, a knife, or whatever happened to be in his hand at the time. The seriousness of this behavior was reflected in the fact that staff were discouraged and seemed unable to continue their efforts because of a sense of failure, frustration, and resentment attributable to this person's disruption of the overall program. Further, they felt that this behavior was unpredictable and, as a result, doubly dangerous. Other evidence of the social validity of this problem was that the State Department of Mental Health had taken the position that if the problem could not be rapidly resolved, the person was going to be removed and placed in a state institution.

Past Treatment

When this person was younger, a national expert was consulted to develop a treatment program. The main thrust of the intervention at that time was overcorrection, which was successful in suppressing the behavior for a period of time. However, as he got older and bigger, this was no longer a practical intervention strategy and it had to be discontinued because of the staff's concerns for their safety. They and we also attempted to solve this problem with fairly sophisticated and carefully designed schedules of reinforcement. However, this approach also failed. It was at this point that a comprehensive assessment was initiated.

Functional Analysis

The analysis identified two situations that were clearly discriminative for this behavior. One category involved delays, such as when he was asked to wait for something that he wanted (e.g., a reinforcer or a desired activity). A second category of antecedents involved interruptions of his routines. In fact, these kinds of antecedents accounted for approximately 85% of his aggressive behavior.

Treatment Program

The four-part intervention program included an *ecological component*, in which staff developed a comprehensive, 15-minute-by-15-minute structured schedule for him for the entire day. This schedule was communicated to him concretely through a sequence of pictures to which he was oriented at each change in activity. A token economy also was established to help motivate him through this schedule of activities. Further, staff planned for a diversity of tasks in settings involving functional and chronologically age appropriate activities.

Positive programming involved discrete trial to strengthen instructional control using differential reinforcement for compliance to staff requests to engage in a variety of activities. In addition, discrete trial and free operant shaping was designed to give him a greater tolerance for situations involving delays and interruptions. For example, the beginning of a discrete trial was to say, "Would you please wait for your French fries? Don't they look delicious? Would you please wait for them? [brief pause] Thank you for waiting for them. Here they are. You may eat them now." Staff scheduled five discrete trials a day in which the subject was asked to wait longer and longer periods for a variety of favored reinforcers. When the delay was long enough, staff also inserted requests to engage in certain tasks and activities (e.g., setting the table, sweeping the floor, etc.). The key here was errorless training and only gradually increasing the requirement. Free operant shaping was also implemented parallel with the discrete trial shaping (i.e., staff were to catch him waiting spontaneously for this brief period of time and to then reinforce him). There was a similar discrete trial and free operant approach to teaching him to tolerate interruptions in his routines. Finally, staff used communication training to teach him to label his emotions, his frustrations and feelings about having to wait or having something interrupted.

For *direct treatment*, there was a continuation of some of the progressive DRO schedules that had been in place in the past but that had not by themselves been effective in reducing the problem. The staff felt that these were important in terms of giving him some positive reinforcement and feedback for his success on a daily and progressive basis. For *reactive strategies*, when he was aggressive the goal was immediate control over the problem. If he were firmly told to sit down or to go somewhere when he was being aggressive, he would listen 50% of the time. Another 35 or 40% of the time, the problem could be dealt with by utilizing a combination of redirection and interpositioning an object such as a sofa pillow between him and the mediator as he was being redirected. Occasionally those methods failed and a state approved system of physical management had to be used to prevent injury. This occurred in the beginning of intervention and was virtually unnecessary toward the end.

Results

Figure 2 presents 4-week blocks of data for 200 weeks. It portrays the cumulative frequency of aggressive acts over this period of time. During baseline, the slope represents an average rate of approximately 1.71 episodes per week. To mediate the treatment program, we recommended an intensive intervention team (Donnellan, LaVigna, Zambito, & Thvedt, 1985). The first phase of treatment was therefore implemented by a 1:1 intervention team. During that phase of intervention, there was an average rate of occurrence of 0.61 times per week, a more than 50% decrease from baseline. The second phase of intervention was implemented by the regular group home staff without any special staff in the home environment. During this phase, the average rate of occurrence was 0.26 times per week. During a 3-month follow-up period, the behavior occurred only once. This represents a rate of 0.08 times per week.

To summarize, there was an immediate two-thirds reduction. The durability of treatment effects is reflected in that there was continuing reduction over the 4-year period of treatment and follow-up. Data were collected 24 hours a day across all settings. No formal measures have been taken of side effects, so we cannot formally report whether there were any side effects associated with this treatment. In terms of social validity, however, this person currently participates in all activities scheduled in the community (e.g., grocery shopping, bowling, eating out, banking, etc.) and he has been placed in a supported employment position in the community. In fact, group home staff now feel that he should have the same access to the community as do the others who live in the home, and many now prefer his company to the company of others.

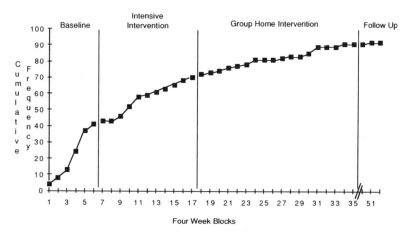

FIGURE 2: Cumulative record of aggressive episodes.

CONCLUSIONS

In conclusion, there seem to be a number of implications of positive programming. The first is that positive programming offers promise for producing the durable treatment effects that have been so elusive with other behavior reduction strategies. It does so because it is based on an analysis of the role the aberrant behavior serves the person and aims to establish a new behavioral repertoire that legitimizes that role and teaches the person more effective and more socially acceptable ways of dealing with the environment. A second implication is that no single treatment procedure, including a positive program, is likely to be fully effective by itself, requiring instead multielement treatment packages. It may be that it is only through the careful design of complex treatment packages that we can accomplish socially valid, rapid, durable, and generalized treatment effects without negative side effects.

This discussion of positive programming also has implications for the use of aversive procedures in behavioral treatment. Clearly, aversive procedures do not teach adaptive behavior. As a result, as a sole strategy and at best, they may produce only short term suppression. As part of a treatment package, aversive procedures may also be contraindicated because they may produce effects that interfere with positive programming, such as elicited aggression. Further, the use of punishment may preclude access to environments that are necessary for a full application of positive programming strategies.

There is increasing concern about the field's possible overuse, misuse, and abuse of aversive procedures. This concern is reflected in the recent positions taken against aversive treatment by leading professional and advocacy organizations such as The Association for Persons with Severe Handicaps (TASH) and the Association for Retarded Citizens (ARC). It is also reflected in increasing legislation and regulation at federal, state, and agency levels. However, the largest implication of this concern for professional practice may not be for sanctions against the use of aversive procedures. Rather, standards may more importantly have to address mandatory requirements for positive programming, the sophisticated instructional techniques that are often required for their implementation, ecological manipulation strategies, nonaversive direct treatment strategies, reactive strategies, and the assessment strategies on which these approaches are based.

The researcher's role is clear: to further develop and validate treatment procedures that demonstrably improve the quality of life and full community presence and participation for all individuals, regardless of handicapping condition or associated problem behaviors.

REFERENCES

Association for the Advancement of Behavior Therapy Task Force Report (1982). The treatment of self-injurious behavior. *Behavior Therapy, 13,* 529–554.

Adams, G. L., Tallon, R. J., & Stangl, J. M. (1980). Environmental influences on self-stimulatory behavior. *American Journal of Mental Deficiency, 85,* 171–175.

Ayllon, T. (1963). Intensive treatment of psychotic behavior by stimulus satiation and food reinforcement. *Behavior Research and Therapy, 1,* 53–61.

Azrin, N. H. (1958). Some effects of noise on human behavior. *Journal of the Experimental Analysis of Behavior, 1,* 183–200.

Brown, L., Nietupski, J., & Homre-Nietupski, S. (1976). The criterion of ultimate functioning and public school services for severely handicapped students. In L. Brown, N. Certo, & T. Crowner (Eds.), *Papers and programs related to public school services for secondary age severely handicapped students.* (Vol. VI, Part 1, pp. 1–12). Madison, WI: Madison Metropolitan School District.

Carr, E. G., & Durand, V. M. (1985). Reducing behavior problems through functional communication training. *Journal of Applied Behavior Analysis, 18,* 111–126.

Cautela, J. R., & Groden, J. (1978). *Relaxation: A comprehensive manual for adults, children, and children with special needs.* Champaign, IL: Research Press.

Davidson, P. W., Kleene, B. M., Carroll, M., & Rockowitz, R. J. (1983). Effects of naloxone on self-injurious behavior: A case study. *Applied Research in Mental Retardation, 4,* 1–4.

Donnellan, A. M. (1980). An educational perspective of autism: Implications, curriculum development and personnel preparation. In B. Wilcox & A. Thompson (Eds.), *Critical issues in educating autistic children and youth.* Washington, DC: U.S. Department of Education, Office of Special Education.

Donnellan, A. M., Kosovac, L., & Clark, M. J. (in press). *Mediating behavior challenges presented by individuals with dual sensory impairments.* Seattle, WA: The Association for Persons with Severe Handicaps, Technical Assistance Project.

Donnellan, A. M., LaVigna, G. W., Negri-Shoultz, N., & Fassbender, L. L. (1988). *Progress without punishment.* New York: Teachers College Press.

Donnellan, A. M., LaVigna, G. W., Zambito, J., & Thvedt, J. (1985). A time limited intensive intervention program to support community placement for persons with severe behavior problems. *Journal of the Association for Persons with Severe Handicaps, 10*(3), 123–131.

Donnellan, A. M., & Mirenda, P. L. (1983). A model for analyzing instructional components to facilitate generalization for severely handicapped students. *Journal of Special Education, 17,* 319–331.

Donnellan, A. M., Mirenda, P. L., Mesaros, R. A., & Fassbender, L. L. (1984). Analyzing the communicative functions of aberrant behavior. *Journal of the Association for Persons with Severe Handicaps, 3,* 201–212.

Egel, A. L., Richman, G.S., & Koegel, R. L. (1981). Normal peer models and autistic children's learning. *Journal of Applied Behavior Analysis, 14,* 3–12.

Foxx, R. M., & Livesay, J. (1984). Maintenance of response suppression following overcorrection: A 10-year retrospective examination of eight cases. *Analysis and Intervention of Developmental Disabilities, 4,* 65–80.

Gordon, T. (1970). *Parent effectiveness training.* New York: P. H. Wyden.

Groden, J., & Cautela, J. R. (1984). Use of imagery procedures with students labeled "trainable retarded." *Psychological Reports, 54,* 595–605.

Horner, R. D. (1980). The effects of an environmental "enrichment" program on the behavior of institutionalized profoundly retarded children. *Journal of Applied Behavior Analysis, 13,* 473–491.

Kanfer, F. H., & Saslow, G. (1969). Behavioral diagnosis. In C. M. Franks (Ed.), *Behavior therapy: Appraisal and status.* New York: McGraw-Hill.

Koegel, R. L., Dunlap, G., & Dyer, K. (1980). Intertrial interval duration and learning in autistic children. *Journal of Applied Behavior Analysis, 13,* 91–99.

LaVigna, G. W. (1983). The Jay Nolan Center: A community-based program. In E. Schopler & G. B. Mesibou (Eds.), *Autism in adolescents and adults.* New York: Plenum Publishing Corporation.

LaVigna, G. W. (1987). The case against aversive stimuli: A review of the clinical and empirical evidence. An invited paper presented at the 13th Annual Convention of the Association for Behavior Analysis, May 25-28, 1987, Nashville, TN.

LaVigna, G. W., & Donnellan, A. M. (1986). *Alternatives to punishment: Solving behavior problems with non-aversive strategies.* New York: Irvington Publishers.

Lozoff, B., & Brittenham, G. M. (1986). Behavioral aspects of iron deficiency. *Progress in Hematology, 16,* 23–53.

Mirenda, P. L., & Donnellan, A. M. (1987). Issues in curriculum development. In D. J. Cohen & A. M. Donnellan (Eds.), *Handbook of autism and pervasive developmental disorders* (pp. 211–226). New York: John Wiley.

Mizuno, T., & Yugari, Y. (1974). Self-mutilation in the Lesch-Nyhan syndrome. *Lancet, 1,* 76.

Palotai, A., Mance, A., & Negri, N. A. (1982). *Averting and handling aggressive behavior.* Columbia, SC: South Carolina Department of Mental Health.

Piaget, J., & Inhelder, B. (1969). *The psychology of the child.* New York: Basic Books.

Rago, W. V., Jr., Parker, R. M., & Cleland, C. C. (1978). Effects of increased space in the social behavior of institutionalized profoundly retarded male adults. *American Journal of Mental Deficiency, 82,* 554–558.

Rhodes, W. C. (1967). The disturbing child: A problem of ecological management. *Exceptional Children, 33,* 449–455.

Russo, D. C., Cataldo, M. F., & Cushing, P. J. (1981). Compliance training and behavioral covariation in the treatment of multiple problems. *Journal of Applied Behavior Analysis, 14,* 209–222.

Schwartz, A., Goldiamond, I., & Howe, M. W. (1975). *Social casework: A behavioral approach.* New York: Columbia University Press.

Schlinger, H., & Blakely, E. (1987). Function-altering effects of contingency-specifying stimuli. *The Behavior Analyst, 10,* 41–45.

Stokes, T. F., & Baer, D. M. (1977). An implicit technology of generalization. *Journal of Applied Behavior Analysis, 10,* 349–367.

Strain, P. S. (1983). Generalization of autistic children's social behavior change: Effects of developmentally integrated and segregated settings. *Analysis and Intervention in Developmental Disabilities, 3,* 23–34.

Sulzer-Azaroff, B., & Mayer, G. R. (1977). *Behavior modification procedures for school personnel.* Hinsdale, IL: The Dryden Press, Inc.

Touchette, P. (1983). *Nonaversive amelioration of SIB by stimulus control transfer.* Paper presented at the Annual Convention of the American Psychological Association, August 26-30, 1983, Anaheim, CA.

Touchette, P. E., MacDonald, R. F., & Langer, S. N. (1985). A scatter plot for identifying stimulus control of problem behavior. *Journal of Applied Behavior Analysis, 18,* 343–351.

Willis, T. J., & LaVigna, G. W. (1983). *Emergency management guidelines.* Los Angeles: Institute for Applied Behavior Analysis.

Willis, T. J., LaVigna, G. W., & Donnellan, A. M. (1987). *Behavior assessment guide.* Los Angeles: Institute for Applied Behavior Analysis.

Winterling, V., & Dunlap, G. (1987). The influence of task variation on the aberrant behaviors of autistic students. *Education and Treatment of Children, 10,* 105–119.

Wolpe, J. (1973). *Psychotherapy by reciprocal inhibition.* Stanford, CA: Stanford University Press.

Zivolich, S., & Thvedt, J. (1983). *Assault crisis training: Prevention and intervention.* Huntington Beach, CA: Special Education Counseling Service.

Behavioral Diagnostics

Jon S. Bailey
and
David A. M. Pyles

Behavior Management Consultants, Inc.
and Florida State University

Carrie, a 23-year-old woman with severe retardation, tears at her face causing deep abrasions and must be restrained to prevent her from doing severe tissue damage. Tom, a 29-year-old man with profound retardation, throws himself from his wheelchair, causing massive contusions to his face and head. It is proposed that he be strapped in his chair so that he cannot get out. Melissa, a 35-year-old woman with profound retardation, bangs her head so severely that her physician is considering giving her a powerful psychotropic medication. Walter, a 33-year-old man with severe retardation, has severe and unpredictable tantrums, in which he will attack others and occasionally himself. Debbie, a 25-year-old woman with severe retardation, cries, sobs and screams loudly and at length. It is assumed that she is trying to get attention, so she is sent to the corner of the room by herself.

These cases and a host of others have confronted us over the past 5 years, straining the limits of our knowledge of behavior analysis. Thankfully, there is a prohibition in Florida against the use of "noxious or painful stimuli" in the treatment of retarded citizens. Partly as a result of the prohibition, and somewhat by accident, we have been forced to examine the factors that might be causing these severely disruptive, aggressive, and self-injurious behaviors to occur.

The now common expression "Behavior is a function of its consequences" resulted from Skinner's early laboratory research (Skinner, 1938) and was subsequently developed into a full scale system for understanding human behavior (Skinner, 1953). This model has stimulated unprecedented applied research (Bailey, Shook, Iwata, Reid, & Repp, 1986) and clinical application and has become the major treatment mode for persons with developmental disabilities in the United States. There can be no doubt that this movement has helped these persons in significant ways. However, it seems that such widespread success can lead to a narrow perspective. Practitioners of behavior analysis may come to believe that *all* behavior is a function of its consequences, thus leading them to ignore or discount other possible causative factors. Our work, for example, has shown us that a variety of physical, environmental, and medical circumstances can greatly increase the likelihood that severe tantrums, aggression, and self-injurious behavior will occur—factors *unrelated* to the *consequences* of the behavior.

THE MEDICAL MODEL

The medical model is generally discounted by the typical behavior analyst. One conjures up visions of Freud explaining complex behavioral phenomena by inventing inner psychic processes that produce just such effects. There is, of course, another medical model, the one we all encounter when we visit our family physician with an ailment or illness. Basically, the contemporary physician will ask a series of questions, and run a few lab tests, to determine the cause of the malady. He or she will want to determine something about your recent history of other illnesses, exposure to hazardous environments, possible allergies, any changes in life style, and so on. Based on this diagnostic process, the physician will make a guess as to the likely cause of your ailment and proceed to prescribe a course of treatment (ranging from simple bedrest to prescription medication to possible surgery). It is upon *this* medical model that our *behavioral diagnostic* approach is based.

ACTIVE VERSUS PASSIVE
BEHAVIOR MANAGEMENT

There is a natural tendency to resist the introduction of new terminology; however, in this case we believe it is warranted. The terms we use can guide our actions, and if new terminology does so more effectively, it should be welcomed. In this case, we believe there is a more effective way of looking at the factors affecting behavior than the traditional, consequence-oriented, operant model.

In the operant model, the three-term contingency is the basis for explaining behavioral phenomena. Perhaps for historical reasons, the emphasis has been on the third term: the *consequences* of behavior. A response is said to occur in the presence of a stimulus, and is followed by consequences, determining the probability of future occurrence. The role of the S^D, or antecedent stimulus, is subordinate to the S^{R+}, or consequence (in this case a reinforcer).

Manipulating the consequences of behavior in order to change the future probability of occurrence is the major endeavor of many behavior analysts. Using our proposed terminology, we would refer to this approach as *active behavior management* (i.e., changing the behavior by *acting* upon it, i.e., following it with a planned consequence).

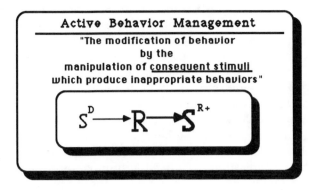

FIGURE 1: Active behavior management.

If, on the other hand, a behavior occurred because of an *antecedent* stimulus, and it were possible to modify the behavior by changing *that* event, we would label it as *passive* behavior management (i.e., changing the behavior *without* directly acting upon it). In the simplest case, if it were possible to prevent the (aversive) stimulus from occurring, precluding the response, it would not be necessary to manipulate the *consequences* of the behavior at all.

It is probably desirable to use passive behavior management strategies whenever they are indicated. While it might be possible to change a behavior that is a result of some antecedent condition using consequence manipula-

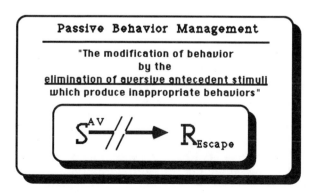

FIGURE 2: Passive behavior management.

tions (e.g., you could punish someone for sneezing in the presence of pepper), it is clearly unethical and may be less than effective. Changing the antecedent environment can be relatively easy, requiring little staff training and minimal monitoring. Passive strategies, as we shall see, generally are easily established and maintained. The question then becomes, "How do we know when to use each approach?" Again, with our new terminology, we would argue that the first step for the behavior analyst is to perform a functional analysis or, in our terms, a *behavioral diagnosis*, to determine the factors causing the behavior to occur. Once this diagnosis has taken place, it should be obvious whether the active or the passive behavior management strategy is most appropriate for the case at hand. There is a small body of research employing the diagnostic approach (although the term is not used), establishing the foundation for this method.

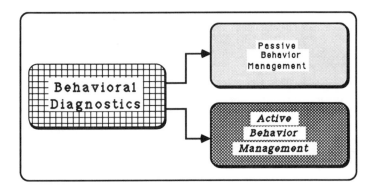

FIGURE 3: Behavioral diagnostics.

EXPERIMENTAL FOUNDATIONS
FOR BEHAVIORAL
DIAGNOSTICS

There are currently several means available for determining probable causes of behavior. The primary ones involve performing an analysis by constructing analogue situations to natural environments; performing a pattern analysis; hypothesis testing; and using a computer to analyze environmental variables.

Functional Analysis via Analogue Situations

Lovaas, Freitag, Gold, & Kassorla (1965) first used analogue situations to determine the cause of self-injury. Since then other researchers (Iwata, Dorsey, Slifer, Bauman, & Richman, 1982; Mace & Knight, 1986; Mace, Page, Ivancic, & O'Brien, 1986; Parrish, Iwata, Dorsey, Bunck, & Slifer, 1985) have used similar methodologies to ascertain functional variables of aberrant behaviors.

The basic procedure is to construct situations that mimic naturally occurring environments. Thus, to test whether the behavior is maintained by attention, one would construct the therapy session so that attention was provided contingent on the occurrence of inappropriate responding. To test whether demands are responsible, the therapist places demands on the client and terminates them contingent upon inappropriate responding.

One caution in using analogue settings: they can be labor intensive and time consuming. Enough sessions of each condition must be run so that stable rates are obtained; personnel must be able to run sessions without interruptions, and so forth. However, the data obtained from performing a functional analysis are very useful in determining variables responsible for the occurrence of maladaptive behaviors.

Pattern Analysis

Another means of determining the causes of maladaptive behavior is to perform a pattern analysis. Pattern analyses are useful "when the target behavior is frequent, and informal observations do not suggest a reliable correspondence with anything in particular" (Touchette, MacDonald, & Langer, 1985).

To perform a pattern analysis, make a scatterplot by dividing the day into at least half-hour intervals on the ordinate and divide a month into its respective days on the abscissa. Then, when a targeted behavior occurs, a mark is placed in the box corresponding to the date and time. Different types of marks can be used to indicate varying frequencies within intervals. If a pattern is established, examine the differences between environments where the problematic behavior occurs and those where it does not. Then, systematically eliminate variables until the operative one is determined.

Using a scatterplot to determine patterns of responding is the easiest method of collecting data to determine causative variables. It is not difficult to set up or to train staff to use. However, the data obtained are correlational and not causative; further analysis is necessary to determine the actual variables that are responsible.

Hypothesis Testing

Another means of determining functional variables is by setting up a series of short experiments. In this approach, the practitioner treats the behavior as if it were caused by a given event; s/he designs an intervention that corresponds to one of the major usual causative variables during a given session. Thus, extinction would be used during a positive reinforcement session, compliance training during a negative reinforcement session, and so on, until all major hypotheses are tested.

Repp, Felce, and Barton (1988) used this procedure to determine the causative variables for stereotypic and self-injurious behaviors. By testing the possible variables, they were able to determine the function of the targeted behaviors and select one best treatment. This approach is very similar to the analogue settings approach, except that the treatment was used to determine the operative factors rather than presentation of the variable itself. Thus, rather than allowing a demand to result in escape (analogue setting), a compliance training program would be used (hypothesis testing).

This procedure can also be very time consuming and labor intensive to perform. However, like analogue settings, the data obtained are extremely useful for designing effective treatments based on the functional variables.

Computer Analysis

The advent of microcomputers brings possibilities for analyzing the setting events and stimulus control factors not previously possible. Large amounts of data can be entered into a computer and analyzed very quickly; unusual combinations of stimulus settings and events can be determined that all too human practitioners could very easily overlook.

Gardner, Souza, Scabbia, and Breuer (1985) used a microcomputer (Kaypro 4) to analyze a client's aggressive behavior. The client had received traditional behavior management techniques, psychotropic medications, and confinement to an intensive behavioral shaping program, all without success. His behavior was analyzed according to variables such as intensity, frequency, day of week by class assignment, location of aggression, family visits, and passage of his physical biorhythm through the midline stage (indicating a general weakening of his condition), to name but a few of them.

These data were entered into the computer and correlations computed. The probability of an aggressive episode was 0.83 when the following conditions were in effect: his biorhythm was passing through the midline and his weight was decreasing; he was receiving a visit from his family;

and following the visit, was being introduced into a highly structured environment. Without this confluence of conditions, the probability of aggression was 0.14.

The treatment designed involved reducing the amount of structure following family visits. This intervention decreased the probability of an aggressive episode following a family visit to 0.33 during the first 3 months of intervention, followed by a decrease to 0.00 during the next 3 months (Gardner, Souza, et al., 1985).

Gardner, Souza, et al. (1985) also used similar procedures to determine that self-injurious behaviors were caused by seasonal allergies for one client; antihistamines were prescribed whenever an episode of self-abuse occurred, reducing the frequency during outbreaks from nearly constantly to less than 5 minutes per day.

Gardner, Swanson, Sutton, and Breuer (in press) did a cost-benefit analysis comparing the use of microcomputers with traditional means for performing biannual behavioral assessments. They found that the cost of using the microcomputer to analyze and assess the client's behavior, write reports, and so forth, was approximately one-fourth that of using a psychologist, clerk, or other personnel to do the same work. Furthermore, the computer generated reports were consistently judged superior to those of the psychologist by direct care staff, program management, and client advocates.

Thus, the use of computers holds great promise for the diagnosis of aberrant behaviors. The increase in memory capacities and falling price per kilobyte of data make the promise of computer diagnosis of behaviors even greater for the future.

BASIC DIAGNOSTIC
QUESTIONS

We have discussed the multiple causation of behavior and means of analyzing behavior so that we can begin to determine the functions the targeted behaviors serve. Based on the variables discussed, we have designed a list of questions to ask when addressing any behavior referred for treatment.

Situational Variables/Setting Events

• *Are there any circumstances under which the behavior does NOT occur?* An affirmative answer to this question demonstrates the behavior is under some sort of stimulus control and that the problem could be prevented by eliminating the circumstance/event. What are the features of this environ-

BEHAVIORAL DIAGNOSIS and TREATMENT INFORMATION FORM

Client _____ Target Behavior _____

1. Situational Variables/Setting Events

Is there any circumstance under which the behavior does NOT occur?

Is there any circumstance under which the behavior ALWAYS occurs?

Does it occur at certain times of the day?

Does the behavior occur only with certain people?

Could the behavior be related to any skills deficit?

Recommendations

2. Physiological Variables

Does the behavior occur during certain seasons of the year?

Could the behavior be the result of any form of discomfort (i.e., an escape response to headache, stomach ache, dizziness, blurred vision, or ear infection, etc.)?

Could the client be signalling some deprivation condition (e.g., thirst, hunger, lack of rest, etc.)?

Could the behavior be a side-effect of medication (e.g., tired, unsteady, thirsty, confused, sick to the stomach, buzzing in ears, toxic levels of medication, etc.)?

Could the behavior be caused by allergies (e.g., food, materials in the environment)?

Recommendations

3. Operant Variables

Does the behavior allow the client to gain attention?

Does the behavior allow the client to escape the training situation?

Does behavior occur to compete with boredom or loneliness?

Does the behavior provide self-stimulation activity?

Does the behavior occur collateral with any other behavior or as part of a chain of behavior?

Does the behavior occur as a result of having another ongoing behavior terminated?

Recommendations

4. Other

Does the client have any identified reinforcers?

Does the behavior cause serious tissue damage?

Does the behavior have any serious negative effects on training?

Recommendations

FIGURE 4: Behavioral diagnosis and treatment information form.

ment that do *not* occasion/reinforce the maladaptive behavior? One client always banged his head when he was in his wheelchair; when he was taken out and placed on a mat, the headbanging stopped.

● *Are there any circumstances under which the behavior always occurs?* If so, compare the problematic environment with the one where the problem does *not* occur. What are the differences between these two environments? After determining discrepancies between the two, systematically eliminate variables until the one(s) maintaining responding are discovered. Another client always began self-abusing when being prepared for a bath in the morning; when bathing was shifted to the evening, the self-abuse almost completely stopped.

• *Does the behavior occur at certain times of the day?* A scatterplot is used to answer this question. Examine times the behaviors consistently occur. Are they most likely during shift change, or before meals? If so, change the environment, gradually fading in the problematic components until they do not occasion the behavior. We have observed many clients engage in agitated and aggressive behavior around mealtimes. When they are fed first, or get part of their meal (e.g., milk) while waiting, the agitation subsides.

• *Does the behavior occur only with certain people?* Scatterplots can help provide this information. If a large percentage of the behaviors occurs when a certain person is working, examine that person's interaction style with the client. He or she could be too abrupt with the client or reinforce inappropriate behavior, or there could be some not easily discernible feature of that person causing the client to react.

• *Could the behavior be related to any skills deficit?* Many people with severe or profound developmental disabilities are unable to communicate verbally. Thus, they cannot say a task is too difficult, not stimulating enough, or they are sick and should be left alone. Examine the types of demands made on the client, and look for patterns across tasks (e.g., ones the client is performing consistently below criterion). Try varying the types of tasks more frequently to increase stimulation. If the behavior is a result of a skill deficit, the best approach is to teach an appropriate response, a means of communication, or other skills.

Physiological Variables

• *Does the behavior occur during certain seasons of the year?* If so, one possible explanation could be allergies. Does the behavior occur mostly when there is a lot of dust or pollen in the air? Examining graphs across months of the year can provide information about seasonal variables. Also checking the medical records for allergies, asthma, and so forth is very helpful in pinpointing these types of problems.

• *Could the behavior be the result of any form of discomfort (i.e., an escape response to headache, stomachache, dizzy, blurred vision, ear infection, etc.).* If the behavior has been stable and low frequency, and suddenly increases with no identifiable environmental change, determine whether the client has become ill. Examine nurse's notes and physician's orders and compare to the graphs to determine a correlation between illness/discomfort and outbreaks of aggression, self-injurious behaviors, or other inappropriate acts.

• *Could the client be signalling some deprivation condition (e.g., thirst, hunger, lack of rest, etc.)* Does examination of the problematic environment reveal a regular time of occurrence across days? Is the client simply trying to get a drink and aggresses against staff when blocked? How many hours per night does the client sleep? (Nursing departments often track the amount of sleep clients get.) Examine factors such as these to determine whether some state of deprivation exists. Probe giving naps, drinks, snacks, and so forth. One should treat maladaptive behaviors that are caused by physical discomfort using behavioral interventions only in emergency situations (e.g., when the client is causing tissue or property damage, etc.).

• *Could the behavior be a side effect of medication (e.g., tired, unsteady, thirsty, confused, sick to the stomach, buzzing in ears, toxic levels of the drug)?* If a client is on psychotropic or other medications, work closely with the psychiatrist or physician and the nursing department. Determine the side effects of each drug in the *Physician's Desk Reference* (PDR). Did the behavior begin to occur shortly after beginning a new medication regimen? A client who was poking her ear was found to be responding to a medication that in some patients causes tinnitus. When the medication was changed, the earpoking stopped.

• *Could the behavior be caused by allergies (e.g., food, materials in the environment, etc.)?* As noted earlier, allergies can occasion aggression, self-injurious behaviors, and so on. Examine medical records, seasonal fluctuations in behavior, other signs of allergies. Unfortunately, Medicare/Medicaid does not usually pay for allergy tests; thus, this cause of behavior could be easily overlooked. Itching, scratching, tearing at his/her clothes may be the result of allergic reactions.

Operant Variables

• *Does the behavior allow the client to gain attention?* Does the client wait for staff to look before engaging in a maladaptive behavior? Attention provided contingently maintains maladaptive behaviors such as aggression and self-injurious behaviors. If attention is maintaining the behavior, the appropriate treatment is differential reinforcement for appropriate behavior and/or extinction (if feasible) for the inappropriate behavior.

• *Does the behavior allow the client to escape the training situation?* Do training demands cause the onset of tantrums, stereotypic, or self-injurious behaviors? If so, the client must be shaped to comply to requests without showing serious behavior problems. Time-out is *not* the treatment of choice—it only reinforces escape behavior.

• *Does the behavior occur to compete with loneliness or boredom?* Does the targeted response occur when the client is not engaged in other behaviors or when other people or activities/materials are not accessible? If so, the client's schedule should be enriched—either by making activities available or by engaging in them with the client. Sometimes, s/he must be trained in appropriate use of the materials. Consequating behaviors caused by boredom without providing appropriate materials is unethical, and will most likely result in the program's failure.

• *Does the behavior provide self-stimulation activity?* Some behaviors are reinforcing in and of themselves. Participating in sports, reading, or involvement in hobbies are examples of acceptable stimulation activities in the "normal" population. Because persons with developmental disabilities have limited behavioral repertoires, self-reinforcing activities often take the form of self-stimulatory behaviors. These behaviors often occur more frequently when the client has no access to appropriate activities, materials, or people.

• *Does the behavior occur collaterally with any other behavior or as part of a chain of behavior?* Can you see the client escalate in intensity until the target behavior occurs? If so, the whole chain of behaviors and the collateral behaviors must be analyzed, not just the targeted response. Often, it is possible to reduce problematic behaviors by addressing a behavior early in the chain.

• *Does the behavior occur as a result of having another ongoing behavior terminated?* Often requests to terminate an ongoing behavior (e.g., "Stop playing and come inside for a bath") can result in tantrums, aggression, or other maladaptive responses. This set of behaviors is extinction produced. It is important that these maladaptive reactions not result in retracting the request; capitulation would positively reinforce the inappropriate responses.

Other

• *Does the client have any identified reinforcers?* This is an important question to answer. If the client has no known reinforcers, training will be difficult, if not impossible. So will differentially reinforcing other incompatible behaviors. Some states have guidelines against using aversive stimuli without providing an opportunity for reinforcement.

• *Does the behavior cause serious tissue damage?* If so, then it is more urgent to get the behavior under control. The safety of the clients and staff is of utmost importance. Sometimes emergency procedures must be implemented until the controlling variables are known and can be addressed to reduce the possibility of injury. If the behavior does not cause any tissue damage, it may be most appropriate to simply leave it be. Headweaving, some handmouthing, minor motor movements, and noises are often best left untreated.

• *Does the behavior have any serious negative effects on training?* If the behavior is so disruptive that training the client is difficult or impossible, then it must be dealt with. However, in our experience, many "behavior problems" do not affect training adversely. Problems such as stereotypies, while seeming disruptive, quite often cease when clients are presented with interesting, age-appropriate activities or materials and rich schedules of reinforcement for engagement. If a behavior does not actually prevent training, it is possible to simply ignore it and work around it. Attempting to reduce such a behavior, especially using restrictive or aversive procedures, may actually make the problem worse and ultimately prove to be of little benefit to the client.

ISSUES AND IMPLICATIONS

Practical Issues

There are several important practical implications of a behavioral diagnostic approach. For example, the way in which behavioral personnel are trained would change. Instruction in behavioral diagnostics would emphasize the analysis of behavior rather than its treatment. Furthermore, antecedent stimuli would be acknowledged as causing behavior; staff would not focus solely on consequent events.

Another practical implication is that the method of data collection would change. Rather than collecting baseline data solely on frequency, duration, and so on, practitioners would also observe the behavior as it occurs to determine situational concomitants. Scatterplots and situational analyses would enhance traditional types of data collection.

Also, a behavioral diagnostic approach would require behavioral practitioners to work closely with the client's physician, psychiatrist, and nursing staff. Improved cooperation among the various departments of institutions could only be beneficial for clients and should result in improved client care.

A final practical implication of a behavioral diagnostic approach is that it is often less work. It is much easier to provide pain relief to a client suffering from menstrual cramps than to put her in time-out for aggression. Doing the analytical work before programming can save much work later implementing (and constantly revising) a program.

Ethical Implications

One way in which behavioral diagnostics would affect the field of behavior analysis is in the way we conceptualize ethical treatment for clients. For example, it no longer is acceptable to use solely operant procedures to reduce all behavior problems. Using time-out or other aversive procedures to punish a person for aggressing when s/he is sick would constitute unethical practice. Ethically, we are bound to determine the causative variable (if known) before implementing treatment.

Another ethical implication of behavioral diagnostics would involve the way we design living environments and schedule activities. With the knowledge of the effects of various setting events such as crowding, demands, and types of activities, we can begin scheduling activities in such a way as to minimize aberrant behaviors. Some clients may need a nap in the morning or afternoon; others may need a shortened class schedule, and so on.

Finally, we are ethically bound to individualize schedules, analyses, and treatment programs for each client as much as possible. For some clients, we may allow brief periods of stereotypic responding if we have no better activities for them at the time. Given the role that sensory stimulation plays in much of stereotyped behaviors, attempting to reduce them without providing other means of stimulation could be questioned.

Theoretical Implications

The major theoretical implication of a behavioral diagnostics approach is that our understanding of human behavior would change. No longer can we justify a consequence-only explanation of behavior. We must now place much more emphasis on clients' responses to antecedent stimuli, such as dietary restrictions or noise in the environment. For example, if a client aggresses as a result of being placed on a weight reduction diet (given the absence of a life-threatening condition such as diabetes), perhaps we should think twice about imposing our aesthetic values of reasonable appearance on him/her.

RESEARCH ILLUSTRATING
THE "CAUSES" OF
MALADAPTIVE BEHAVIORS

There are three main classes of variables that have been shown to be responsible for maladaptive behaviors: operant variables, such as positive reinforcement, negative reinforcement, and punishment; medical/physiological variables, such as drug side effects, physical discomfort or illness; and setting/situational events, such as the time of day, amount of space available, and the presence of alternative activities to the maladaptive behaviors. The literature review to follow illustrates how each variable has been shown to cause, occasion, or maintain inappropriate behaviors of persons with developmental disabilities.

Operant Variables

Positive Reinforcement

The role of positive reinforcement in the acquisition and maintenance of behavior is well documented in the literature. Indeed, without reinforcers, little, if any, skill acquisition would occur.

Attention provided contingently has been shown to maintain maladaptive responding. Lovaas et al. (1965) demonstrated that a subject's self-destructive behaviors were maintained by the attention she received contingently upon such responding. Iwata et al. (1982) performed a functional analysis of self-injurious behaviors with nine subjects and found that one subject had higher levels of self-abuse when attention was provided contingent upon these behaviors (other subjects had different maintaining variables).

Maladaptive behavior may be reinforcing in and of itself. Wolery, Kirk, and Gast (1985) demonstrated that allowing a subject to engage in 5 seconds of stereotypic responding as a reinforcer resulted in faster skill acquisition than did using verbal praise. Charlop and Kurtz (1987) compared the relative reinforcing salience of stereotypic responding, food, and obsessions (defined as materials the child repetitively requested, searched for, or talked about). Using the "maladaptive" behaviors as reinforcers for training new behaviors, they found that both the obsessions and stereotypic behavior resulted in a higher percentage of correct reponses than did food.

Negative Reinforcement

The role of negative reinforcement in causing aberrant behaviors has been receiving increasing attention. In this paradigm, inappropriate responding functions to escape or avoid an aversive situation. Carr, Newsom, and Binkoff (1976) found that conditions where demands were placed on the subject resulted in greatly higher rates of self-injurious behavior than did free time or the experimenter's making nondemand statements. They used those data to design a treatment embedding the demands in the context of a story. Placing demands in a positive context resulted in 40 times fewer self-hits than did demands alone.

Iwata et al. (1982) demonstrated that in some cases self-injurious behavior can function to escape demands. They designed analogue settings to approximate naturally occurring situations that the subjects encountered. In one condition, attention was provided contingent upon self-injurious behavior. In other conditions, demands were made of the client, or the client was placed in the room alone, and so forth. Iwata et al. found, for some subjects, that a condition where self-injurious behavior terminated demands for 30 seconds resulted in higher rates of self-destructive behaviors than the other conditions.

Other maladaptive behaviors have been identified as being maintained by negative reinforcement. Escape-induced aggression (Carr & Durand, 1985; Carr, Newsom, & Binkoff, 1980) and stereotypic responding (Durand & Carr, 1987; Repp et al., 1988) have also been reported.

One successful method to decrease demand-related maladaptive behaviors is compliance training (Carr & Durand, 1985; Carr et al., 1980; Durand & Carr, 1987; Repp et al., 1988; Russo, Cataldo, & Cushing, 1981). Another is reducing the aversiveness of the demand situation by embedding it in a positive context, a desensitization procedure (Carr et al., 1976). Time-out is obviously contraindicated in the case of demand-related inappropriate behaviors. Escape behaviors would be positively reinforced by the termination of demands when time-out is implemented.

It is important for practitioners to identify how the environments they create might provide negative reinforcement for inappropriate behaviors (Iwata, 1987). One must examine antecedent as well as consequent events to determine whether the difference between the two provides reduction of aversive stimulation. Iwata argued that, if our training situations and demands made on the clients result in the onset of severely disruptive or dangerous behaviors, we should question "whether or not our well-intentioned efforts to teach are in our clients' best interest; at the very least, we must question one or more aspects of our teaching technique." (p. 365).

STIMULUS CONTROL/
SETTING EVENTS

To determine the causes of inappropriate behavior, sometimes one must look beyond the relatively discrete antecedent and consequent events. Kantor (1959; cited in Wahler & Fox, 1981) identified "setting factors" as "immediate circumstances" that influenced which of the various stimulus-response relationships would occur. These relationships are determined through past organism-environment interactions, forming the organism's conditioning history. Such setting events consist of environmental events that are more encompassing and complex than the stimulus-response relationships occurring at the time of the behavior's occurrence.

Setting events include the hungry or satiated state of the organism, physiological and medical conditions, and events that may be temporally distant from the occurrence of the behavior in question. An unsatisfactory interaction with a person in the morning may have bearing on an aggressive episode occurring later that day; a poor night's sleep could be a factor in both the unsatisfactory interaction *and* the aggressive episode.

An analysis of setting events necessitates different types of data collection and analysis than are currently commonly used—a more global analysis becomes necessary (Wahler & Fox, 1981). Simple frequency counts are no longer adequate. Other factors that must be considered are medication regimens and their possible side effects, medical and physiological states (already alluded to, and discussed in more detail in a later section of this chapter), the amount of stimulation available in the environment, and so forth.

A brief clinical example should demonstrate the analysis of these factors. One of the authors once had a client referred for stereotypic responding. The client's stereotypy was a repetitive hand movement. Closer examination of the client also revealed abnormal mouth and tongue movements. A review of the client's past medication regimen and medical history showed a long history of psychotropic medication and a diagnosis of tardive dyskinesia. Obviously, using operant procedures to reduce the frequency of this behavior would have been inappropriate.

Stimulus Control

Recent research has begun to examine setting events of problematic behaviors. Touchette et al. (1985) used a scatterplot to analyze maladaptive behaviors. By examining targeted behaviors as they occurred across time and days, the authors were able to determine patterns of assaultive behavior exhibited by a girl with autism. They replaced stimulus conditions associated with high levels of aggression (an interaction of groups and group activities—neither groups nor instruction alone resulted in aggressive outbreaks) with stimulus conditions associated with lower levels.

Touchette et al. then gradually faded the stimulus conditions more closely approximating the problematic environments into her schedule, until she was reintroduced into her regular routine. This assessment and treatment approach reduced her assaultive behaviors from a range of 53 to 82 per week during baseline to once during a 12 month followup.

Touchette et al. also used a scatterplot to identify patterns of environmental events associated with self-injurious behavior in an autistic man. By systematically excluding variables associated with self-abuse, they were able to determine that the behavior occurred mostly in the presence of one specific staff member. The authors were unable to determine any functional interaction differences between that staff member and another working on the same shift.

The problem was eventually solved when the client began attending a workshop; the staff member associated with lower rates of self-injurious behaviors was then scheduled during the afternoons when the client returned home.

Understimulating Environments

The amount of stimulation available in an environment can determine the occurrence of inappropriate behaviors. In some cases, too little stimulation has been implicated in the onset of problematic behaviors; in others, too much stimulation seems to be responsible.

Iwata et al. (1982) demonstrated that understimulating environments occasion maladaptive behaviors. The results of the functional analysis showed that one subject engaged in higher rates of self-injurious behaviors when alone in a room than when in other conditions.

Using a similar methodology to the Iwata et al. (1982) study, Pyles, Reiss, Rankin, and Bailey (1986) found the highest rates of stereotypic responding when the subject was in a room with no materials, and the lowest rates when activities were made available. Finally, Klaber and Butterfield (1968) found that the highest rates corresponded to periods when the clients were brought into an area with no diversionary activities and coerced into remaining still. The presence of more than one environmental event (understimulating environment and demands to remain still) confounds their findings; they did not attempt systematically to determine the operative variable.

Overstimulating Environments

Too much stimulation has also been implicated in problematic behaviors. Hollis (1971) found that increases in volume from 65 dB to 95 dB resulted in concomitant increases in body rocking. Forehand and Baumeister (1970) exposed a subject who engaged in stereotyped rocking to different levels of both visual and auditory stimulation. They found that increasing levels of visual stimulation were correlated with lower levels of rocking and vice versa, apparently supporting the notion of an understimulating environment occasioning such behavior. However, increased levels in the volume of white noise resulted in *higher* levels of rocking than did lower volumes, indicating that too much stimulation can also be responsible for inappropriate behaviors.

One very interesting possibility arising from the Forehand and Baumeister research is that stereotypic behaviors emitted in response to levels of stimulation in the environment could be modality specific. That is, too much stimulation in one sensory modality (e.g., auditory) could result in stereotypies, whereas too little in another (e.g., visual) could have the same result.

Skill Deficits

Another setting event for inappropriate behaviors involves skill deficiencies, most notably communication skill deficits. There is not as much research documenting behavior problems as a function of insufficient communication abilities; however, sketchy as it is, some does exist.

Carr and Durand (1985) found that aggression, tantrums, and self-injurious behaviors were related to either difficult task demands or low levels of attention in four children with developmental disabilities. After determining the operative variable in a given situation, Carr and Durand taught each child a communicative skill functionally related to the maladaptive behavior. That is, the subjects engaging in aberrant responding because of task difficulty were taught to solicit help from the teachers; those whose behaviors were maintained by low levels of attention were taught to request attention appropriately. In the next condition, the subjects were taught the response that was *not* indicated (i.e., ask for help when they were responding to get more attention and vice versa). This phase was a control condition to demonstrate that *any* communication training would not have been effective—only the one functionally related to the behavior. The results demonstrated that, for each subject, only the training related to the subject's skill deficit was effective in reducing the rates of targeted behaviors.

Donellan, Mirenda, Mesaros, and Fassbender (1984) stated that *all* aberrant responses are communicative in function. That is, inherent in all escape responding is the (unspoken) statement, "Leave me alone—I don't want to do that"; clients engaging in maladaptive, attention-seeking responses are crying out, "Somebody pay attention to me!" Donellan et al. called for a functional analysis to determine which variables are in effect for a given behavior, in order to determine the kind of communication training needed. However, one must question whether this unitary explanation of maladaptive responding is appropriate in all circumstances.

MEDICAL/PHYSIOLOGICAL VARIABLES

Although medical and physiological variables technically comprise a subset of setting events (Gardner, Cole, Davidson, & Karan, 1986; Wahler & Fox, 1981), their importance warrants inclusion as a distinct section.

Pain/Discomfort

Much of the work relating physiological and medical bases of inappropriate behavior, especially self-injurious behavior, has come from Brian Iwata (now at the University of Florida) and colleagues at the Johns Hopkins School of Medicine Pediatric Unit. They have found that much of a client's self-injurious behavior occurs when s/he is in pain or physical discomfort.

Engaging in self-injurious behavior when in pain or physical discomfort could serve at least two possible functions: terminating demands or attenuating the pain. An example of pain or discomfort terminating demands in the "normal" population is provided when a person misses work because of illness. Nonverbal people with severe or profound retardation cannot verbally communicate that they, too, are sick and would like to stay home from work; thus, they use "inappropriate" behaviors to achieve that end.

The other way self-injurious could be maintained by discomfort/pain is pain attenuation. Endogenous opiates such as endorphens are released when an organism is exposed to pain, increasing its pain threshold. Cataldo and Harris (1982) provided evidence that these endogenous opiates are as physically addictive as the exogenous opiates, such as heroin and morphine. Addiction to the internally produced opiates becomes a possible maintaining variable for self-injurious behaviors that initially occurred to attenuate pain.

Neurological Variables

Neurological variables have been implicated as causing or maintaining inappropriate behaviors, such as stereotypic and self-injurious behaviors. Organic syndromes, such as Parkinson's disease, cause repetitive movements similar to some stereotypies. Lesch-Nyhan syndrome is characterized by an affected person's chewing off his/her lips and fingers.

There are two interrelated neurological accounts of behavior: developmental and biochemical.

Developmental explanations rely on the effects of isolation or sensory deprivation early in life. Much of the support comes from the animal research literature; the fact that animals reared in isolation engage in higher rates of stereotypies and self-injury is, by now, well known.

Lovaas, Newsom, and Hickman (1987) cited research indicating that cortical stimulation during critical periods of life is necessary for proper neurological development. Differences in brain anatomy have been found between animals that were raised in enriched environments and those reared in isolation. From this perspective, stimulation is as crucial to an organism's development as other, better-known needs, such as nutrition and water. Practitioners must use these possibilities when intervening in some behavior problems.

Lovaas et al. argued that:

"In certain situations, such as during periods of the day when the individual is allowed privacy, or in severely understaffed, barren institutional wards with inadequately trained personnel, punishing self-stimulatory behavior without also teaching and reinforcing appropriate alternatives would seem simply to constitute unnecessary and possibly harmful harrassment, as well as probably being ineffective." (p. 59)

Biochemical factors sometimes play a role in the etiology and maintenance of stereotypic and self-injurious behaviors. The dopamine pathway has been implicated in the onset of amphetamine-induced stereotypies (Lewis & Baumeister, 1982). Substances causing an increase in dopaminergic activity in the striatum will result in increased stereotypies (Cataldo & Harris, 1982).

We have already discussed the role of endogenous opiates in the development and maintenance of self-injurious behavior, especially concerning pain reduction and possible addiction to those substances. Research has shown that administering naloxone, an opiate antagonist, to reduce the pain threshold has resulted in decreases in self-injurious behaviors. While the relationship between biochemistry and behavior is a fledgling science, recent advances such as nuclear resonance tomography and PET scans should make study of brain function and its subsequent role in behavior more accessible to researchers.

Medication/Drug Effects

The side effects of medications (especially psychotropic medications) on maladaptive behaviors have not been well documented in the behavioral research literature. However, perusal of the *Physician's Desk Reference* on drug side effects will often reveal information such as a drug's causing drowsiness, blurred vision, or irritability.

One well-known side effect of long term psychotropic drug use is tardive dyskinesia. Practitioners must monitor the drugs prescribed for their clients for side effects. It is unethical (and, most likely, will be ineffective) to use operant procedures to control responding that is a side effect of some medication regimen.

SUMMARY

The contemporary behavior analyst, to operate ethically and effectively, must be aware of many more factors affecting behavior than simple consequences. Although the literature demonstrating the effectiveness of *active behavior management* is impressive, a compelling argument can be made that a great number of behavior problem seen in individuals with developmental disabilities may be attributable to factors other than consequences. Our experience has been more often than not that physiological, organic, medication, or situational variables are the actual culprits in maladaptive behavior. Individuals with severe or profound retardation may respond to aversive features of their environment by displaying noncompliance, tantrums, aggression, or self-injurious behavior. These antecedents can affect their behavior just as powerfully as can the consequences of their behavior. Behavior analysts must become sensitive to these potential factors and be prepared to employ *behavioral diagnostic strategies* in the search for the causes of maladaptive behavior. Finally, they must be prepared to design rather unconventional *passive behavior management* treatment programs involving the manipulation of the antecedent environment.

In the case of Carrie, from the example at the beginning of this paper, the analysis yielded the hypothesis that her face scratching was a reaction to sinus blockage caused by seasonal allergies. Her treatment involved daily dosages of antihistamines administered by our nurses and subsequent elimination of the scratching. Tom was found to be suffering from "wheelchair fatigue." When he was allowed to recline on other surfaces (e.g., bean bag chair, mat, bolster) on a regular basis, he did not attempt any form of self-injury. Melissa was found to have a severe case of Pre Menstrual Syndrome as well as seizure disorder, and was treated with the appropriate medications. Her headbanging was reduced to a few minor incidents per month. Walter's tantrums on closer inspection seemed part of a chain of behavior leading to seizure-like attacks. Preliminary evidence suggests that when he is treated with phenobarbital the tantrums and aggression disappear. And finally, Debbie was found to be very sensitive to a variety of discomforting events. She would cry, sob, and scream when she was wet, thirsty, hungry, and tired. Changing her regularly, offering her water every hour and extra snacks in the morning as well as short naps in the early afternoon eliminated the crying and sobbing. She now participates with the other clients and seems to enjoy the house activities.

We eagerly anticipate the development of a technology of behavior change based on this approach that will complement the current technology based on the manipulation of consequences of behavior. It is only when all of these factors are taken into account that we will have achieved an appropriate, ethical, and humane (as well as an effective) system of behavior analysis.

REFERENCES

Bailey, J. S., Shook, G. L., Iwata, B. A., Reid, D. H. & Repp, A. C. (Eds.). (1986). *Behavior analysis in developmental disabilities 1968-1985*. Lawrence, KS: Society for the Experimental Analysis of Behavior.

Carr, E. G., & Durand, V. M. (1985). Reducing behavior problems through functional communication training. *Journal of Applied Behavior Analysis, 18*, 111–126.

Carr, E. G., Newsom, C. D., & Binkoff, J. A. (1976). Stimulus control of self-destructive behavior in a psychotic child. *Journal of Abnormal Child Psychology, 4*, 139–153.

Carr, E. G., Newsom, C. D., & Binkoff, J. A. (1980). Escape as a factor in the aggressive behavior of two retarded children. *Journal of Applied Behavior Analysis, 13*, 101–117.

Cataldo, M. F., & Harris, J. (1982). The biological basis for self-injury in the mentally retarded. *Analysis and Intervention in Developmental Disabilities, 2*, 21–39.

Charlop, M. H., & Kurtz, P. F. (1987). *Using aberrant behaviors as reinforcers with autistic children*. Paper presented at the meeting of the Association for Behavior Analysis, Nashville, TN.

Donellan, A. M., Mirenda, P. L., Mesaros, R. A., & Fassbender, L. L. (1984). Analyzing the communicative functions of aberrant behavior. *Journal of the Association for Persons with Severe Handicaps, 9*, 201–212.

Durand, V. M., & Carr, E. G. (1987). Social influences on self-stimulatory behavior: Analysis and treatment application. *Journal of Applied Behavior Analysis, 20*, 119–132.

Forehand, R., & Baumeister, A. A. (1970). The effect of auditory and visual stimulation on stereotyped rocking behavior and general activity of severe retardates. *Journal of Clinical Psychology, 26*, 426–429.

Gardner, W. I., Cole, C. L., Davidson, D. P., & Karan, O. C. (1986). Reducing aggression in individuals with developmental disabilities: An expanded stimulus control, assessment, and intervention model. *Education and Training of the Mentally Retarded, 21*, 3–12.

Gardner, J. M., Souza, A., Scabbia, A., & Breuer, A. (1985). Using microcomputers to help staff reduce violent behavior. *Computers in Human Services, 1*, 53–61.

Gardner, J. M., Swanson, C., Sutton, T., & Breuer, A. (in press). Microcomputer assessment of persons with developmental disabilities: A cost benefit analysis. *Mental Retardation*.

Hollis, J. H. (1971). Body-rocking: Effects of sound and reinforcement. *American Journal of Mental Deficiency, 75*, 642–644.

Iwata, B. A. (1987). Negative reinforcement in applied behavior analysis: An emerging technology. *Journal of Applied Behavior Analysis, 20*, 361–378.

Iwata, B. A., Dorsey, M. F., Slifer, K. J., Bauman, K. E., & Richman, G. S. (1982). Toward a functional analysis of self-injury. *Analysis and Intervention in Developmental Disabilities, 2*, 3–20.

Kantor, J. R. (1959). *Interbehavioral Psychology*. Granville, Ohio: Principia Press.

Klaber, M. M., & Butterfield, E. C. (1968). Stereotyped rocking—A measure of institution and ward effectiveness. *American Journal of Mental Deficiency, 72*, 13–20.

Lewis, M. H., & Baumeister, A. A. (1982). Stereotyped mannerisms in mentally retarded persons: Animal models and theoretical analyses. *International Review of Research in Mental Retardation, 11*, 123–161.

Lovaas, O. I., Freitag, G., Gold, V. J., & Kassorla, I. C. (1965). Experimental studies in childhood schizophrenia: Analysis of self-destructive behavior. *Journal of Experimental Child Psychology, 2*, 67–84.

Lovaas, I., Newsom, C., & Hickman, C. (1987). Self-stimulatory behavior and perceptual reinforcement. *Journal of Applied Behavior Analysis, 20*, 45–68.

Mace, F. C., & Knight, D. (1986). Functional analysis and treatment of severe pica. *Journal of Applied Behavioral Analysis, 19*, 411–416.

Mace, F. C., Page, T. J., Ivancic, M. T., & O'Brien, S. (1986). Analysis of environmental determinants of aggression and disruption in mentally retarded children. *Applied Research in Mental Retardation, 7*, 203–221.

Parrish, J. M., Iwata, B. A., Dorsey, M. F., Bunck, T. J., & Slifer, K. J. (1985). Behavior analysis, program development, and transfer of control in the treatment of self-injury. *Journal of Behavior Therapy and Experimental Psychiatry, 16*, 159–168.

Physician's desk reference (Vol. 42). (1988). Des Moines, IA: Medical Economics Co., Inc.

Pyles, D. A., Reiss, M. L., Rankin, T., & Bailey, J. S. (1986). *Analysis of stereotypic behaviors of a profoundly retarded male*. Paper presented at the meeting of the Florida Association for Behavior Analysis, Orlando, FL.

Repp, A. C., Felce, D., & Barton, L. E. (1988). Basing the treatment of stereotypic and self-abusive behaviors on hypotheses of their causes. *Journal of Applied Behavior Analysis, 21*, 281–289.

Russo, D. C., Cataldo, M. F., & Cushing, P. J. (1981). Compliance training and behavioral covariation in the treatment of multiple behavior problems. *Journal of Applied Behavior Analysis, 14*, 209–222.

Skinner, B. F. (1938). *The behavior of organisms*. New York: Appleton-Century.

Skinner, B. F. (1953). *Science and human behavior*. New York: The Macmillan Company.

Touchette, P. E., MacDonald, R. F., & Langer, S. N. (1985). A scatterplot for identifying stimulus control of problem behavior. *Journal of Applied Behavior Analysis, 18*, 343–351.

Wahler, R. G., & Fox, J. J. (1981). Setting events in applied behavior analysis: Toward a conceptual and methodological expansion. *Journal of Applied Behavior Analysis, 14*, 327–338.

Wolery, M., Kirk, K., & Gast, D. L. (1985). Stereotypic behavior as a reinforcer: Effects and side effects. *Journal of Autism and Developmental Disorders, 15*, 149–161.

Severe Problems

Aggressive and Disruptive Behavior

Jeffrey S. Danforth
University of Massachusetts Medical Center

Ronald S. Drabman
University of Mississippi Medical Center

In 1986, the U.S. District Court in Alabama approved the final settlement of the *Wyatt v. Stickney* lawsuit (Marchetti, 1987). This litigation was propelled by the philosophy of "normalization" (Nirje, 1969; Wolfensberger, 1972), a principle according persons with mental retardation and mental illness educational, social, and habilitation rights identical to those of the rest of society. The results have been community and educational placement of a significant number of individuals.

Aggressive and disruptive behavior is a special issue for families and professionals seeking to help people who have developmental delays to adapt and prosper in less restrictive home, school, and residential settings. Aggressive and disruptive behavior at problemmatic levels results in alterations of the social environment of the client. This behavior can disrupt normal family relationships and restrict social and interpersonal interactions as significant others avoid the offender. Aggression places these persons, their peers, and their caregivers at physical risk. Disruption precludes effective functioning in education and rehabilitation programs, requires considerable staff effort, and may lead to expulsion. Finally, aggressive and disruptive behavior can jeopardize residential and educational placements in mainstream settings and lead to placement in more restrictive settings.

This paper will review the experimental research on treatment programs designed to reduce or replace aggressive and disruptive behavior. Previous reviews detailed early advances (Repp & Brulle, 1981); therefore, the focus here is exclusively on research published in the 1980s. In that manner we hope to have emphasized the most recent trends in this important area of research.

Three categories involving approaches to treatment of aggressive/disruptive behavior are covered: differential reinforcement of other behavior, functional analyses of controlling variables, and punishment.

111

DIFFERENTIAL
REINFORCEMENT OF
OTHER BEHAVIOR

Differential Reinforcement of Other Behavior (DRO) is a schedule that emerged from behavior analysis research that examined the parameters of behavioral contrast (Reynolds, 1961). With a DRO schedule, reinforcement is presented following the nonoccurrence of a target response within a specified interval. DRO schedules do not reinforce nonoccurrence; it is not possible to increase the rate of a response that does not occur. Instead, *DRO* suggests that behavior other than the target response is reinforced, yet very little research has monitored responses other than the undesired target behavior (Poling & Ryan, 1982).

In spite of terminology/process issues, the DRO procedure has a long history of successful research and application. It is the most frequently used element of treatment programs designed to weaken behavior in people with developmental disabilities (Bates & Wehman, 1977). Earlier reviews of the procedure indicated that DRO rapidly weakened disruptive and aggressive behavior emitted by clients with mental retardation, and follow-up data revealed generalization over time. Most researchers provided food or tokens for reinforcement, and DRO intervals were gradually increased as the clients' behavior came under control (Homer & Peterson, 1980; Poling & Ryan, 1982).

Recent analyses have clarified details about variables responsible for effective response suppression. For example, in two experiments Repp, Barton, and Brulle (1983) used a multiple baseline design across subjects and a multiple schedule within subject design to compare (a) reinforcement delivery when the response had not occurred for the entire time interval (*whole interval DRO*) versus (b) reinforcement delivery when the response had not occurred at the moment the DRO interval ended (*momentary DRO;* see Sulzer-Azaroff & Mayer, 1977). Subjects were four 7- and 8-year-old male students who had mild to moderate mental retardation. In each experiment, whole interval DRO was more effective in decreasing mildly disruptive classroom behavior; however, momentary DRO could maintain the suppression once the behavior was weakened. The authors tested the reinforcing effects of various edibles before the intervention began to rule out possible variability in reinforcer potency. Thus, it was clear that momentary DRO's failure was not caused by an ineffective reinforcer.

A follow-up study was done with elementary school students who had severe and profound mental retardation (Barton, Brulle, & Repp, 1986). The results supported the previous finding that momentary DRO can maintain change once behavior has been decelerated with whole interval DRO. It was also noted that momentary DRO reduces the amount of staff time required to monitor the treatment.

Whole interval and momentary DROs have also been used as treatment for inappropriate sexual behavior. A study by Polvinale and Lutzker (1980) indicated the failure of momentary DRO to effectively reduce public genital self-stimulation, inappropriate sexual interactions, and assaultive behavior. Foxx, McMorrow, Fenlon, & Bittle (1986) addressed the issue of DRO as an intervention for sexual behavior in a study designed to eliminate genital stimulation in public by a 16-year-old male (IQ of 21). A whole interval DRO started at 3 minutes. The interval increased each day that the rate of genital stimulation was equal to or lower than the previous day's rate until the interval was 45 minutes. If the boy successfully passed a DRO interval without genital stimulation, he was allowed to engage in stereotypic hand movements that were rewarded with preferred edibles. A multiple baseline design across class periods showed that genital stimulation decreased and remained infrequent as the DRO intervals were lengthened. The overall rate of hand stereotypy remained constant throughout. Eventually, the opportunity to engage in stereotypic hand movements was eliminated and the child received only preferred edibles as a reward for successful DRO intervals. This study contributes to the application of DRO procedures by providing a framework for lengthening DRO intervals. Particularly encouraging was the effectiveness of whole interval DROs in reducing inappropriate genital stimulation, while previously successful treatments relied on punishment for this type of behavior.

A number of other reports have revealed further strengths and applications of DRO procedures. For example, Luiselli (1984; Luiselli & Slocumb, 1983) demonstrated the DRO's applicability to physically disabled, deaf, and visually impaired students with aggressive and destructive behavior. Rather than being restricted to time-related intervals, Cipani (1981) provided tokens and chocolate milk as a function of consecutive spoonfuls of food taken without messy spilling by a 16-year-old female who had severe mental retardation. Friman, Barnard, Altman, & Wolf (1986) illustrated how the parent of a 16-year-old girl who had severe mental retardation could be taught to use DRO in the home to reduce aggressive pinching.

While DRO is an empirically sound procedure, questions remain regarding the process by which response suppression occurs. Little empirical support is available to justify the assumption that the rate of any appropriate behavior is increased during a DRO contingency. Variables that need further study in efforts to enhance the efficacy of DRO include choice of reinforcers, impact of verbal rules and instructions, and standards by which DRO intervals should be increased.

FUNCTIONAL ANALYSES
OF CONTROLLING VARIABLES

A functional analysis examines relationships in which one variable changes systematically according to the value of another.

In contrast to interventions providing consequences contingent on the occurrence or nonoccurrence of specific target behaviors, many researchers have addressed the advantages of functional analyses that examine (a) controlling variables and (b) other behaviors that covary with targeted aggressive and disruptive behaviors.

Controlling Variables

Some experiments have focused on positive and negative reinforcement processes that seem to maintain disruptive behavior.

In one study, Carr, Newsom, and Binkoff (1980; see also Carr & Newsom, 1985) analyzed the aggressive behaviors of two boys. The subjects were Bob, a 14-year-old boy with a Vineland Social Maturity Score of 3.3, and Sam, a 9-year-old boy with a Vineland Score of 2.3. The first experiment served as an assessment condition using a reversal design. A demand condition alternated with a no-demand condition. Demands consisted of requiring Bob to sit in a chair or presenting Sam with a buttoning task. During the demand condition, the rate of aggressive acts toward the adult in the room was high; during no-demands, the rate was near zero. In a subsequent condition, events that were paired with the end of the demand sessions were observed to function as a "safety signal." The safety signal occurred when the experimenter took off the protective gloves that had been paired with the end of Bob's sessions or removed the buttoning board from Sam's sessions. During the safety signal condition, the rate of aggression decreased dramatically. This was contrasted to a condition where demands were eliminated but the gloves and buttoning board remained present, during which the frequency of aggression was quite high. The data showed that (a) the aggressive behavior was negatively reinforced by escape from a demand situation and (b) stimuli paired with the absence of demands would set the occasion for decreased aggression. This latter analysis is consistent with basic research showing decreased rates of escape responding in the presence of stimuli paired with nonaversive events (Azrin, Hake, Holz, & Hutchinson, 1965).

Based on the findings of this assessment study, three treatment strategies to reduce aggressive behavior were examined by Carr et al. (1980). In the first experiment, preferred food and toy reinforcers were identified for Sam and two demand conditions alternated—one with and one without the reinforcers present. The presence of the preferred reinforcers reduced the frequency of aggression substantially. These results suggested that the food and toys reduced the aversiveness of the demand situation, thereby rendering it less reinforcing to escape from it. In a second experiment, two conditions alternated. In one condition Bob was allowed to leave the demand situation following an aggressive response. In the other condition, a tapping response (patting an index finger on the back of his hand) was reinforced as an escape response. Aggression declined steadily when tapping functioned as an escape response from demanding situations. This finding presented the possibility of clinical applications involving shaping and reinforcing alternative, nonaggressive responses to replace aggressive behavior that serves as an escape response.

Despite the decline of aggressive escape responses, Bob continued to tap the back of his hand to escape from demands, thus precluding educational opportunities. This suggests that teaching suitable escape behavior may not be the most desirable therapeutic alternative in training settings. To solve this problem, a third experiment utilized an extinction procedure. The procedure did not allow Bob the opportunity to escape from demands regardless of the intensity or frequency of his aggression. A reversal design was used to compare this with a condition where aggression was followed by a 1-minute escape from the demand. Results showed that extinction nearly eliminated aggression. Unfortunately, an extinction burst consisting of 3 hours of high frequency aggression preceded the decline in aggression, illustrating the questionable applicability of extinction in less restrictive settings.

Another study designed to assess the variables maintaining inappropriate behavior was conducted by Billingsley and Neel (1985). They examined whether inappropriate behaviors interfered with the performance of desired behaviors that served the same function. Subjects were two 8-year-old children, a boy and a girl, performing at the 3-year-old level. Two behaviors emitted by the children resulted in acquisition of food. The inappropriate response was grabbing at food on a plate. A more desirable behavior was pointing at the food. The authors manipulated which response would serve as the reinforced response. In the baseline conditions, the "highly efficient grab response" precluded the need to point to the food. In the experimental condition, pointing to food was to be reinforced. In this condition, if the food were grabbed it was made unavailable to the subjects and their hands were restrained for 15 seconds. If the child pointed, s/he received the food without comment. The results of the experimental condition showed that the pointing response soon replaced grabbing. The authors pointed out that the undesirable behavior was reduced as its function was reduced, illustrating the applicability of functional analyses to the management of disruptive behavior.

The above experiments reveal how analyses of controlling variables can lead directly to therapeutic strategies designed to influence aggressive and disruptive behaviors. The treatment utility of the assessment underscores the quality of the functional analyses (Hayes, Nelson, & Jarrett, 1987).

Response Covariation

Another line of research focused on other behaviors that are functionally related to the targeted disruptive behavior. In general terms, this research examined variables that maintained both the defiant behavior and related appropriate behavior. For example, Russo, Cataldo, & Cushing (1981) studied the relationship between disruptive behavior and compliance to adult commands. Subjects were three children: a 3-year, 7-month male with a Bayley level of 2 years; a 3-year, 6-month boy with a Bayley level of 1.5; and a 5-year-old girl with an IQ of 60. In an analog setting, compliance was measured simultaneously with negative behaviors such as crying, self-injury, aggression, or hair pulling. Two conditions alternated in an ABAB design with each child. In the baseline condition, a standard number of adult requests were presented, but differential reinforcement consequences were not provided. The second condition was identical except that compliance produced small pieces of food intended to reinforce the child's rate of following directions. Results indicated that compliance increased but, in addition, the rate of disruptive behavior (nontarget behavior) decreased. Russo et al. (1981) suggested that these classes of behavior were inverse response classes, "said to exist if a reinforcement contingency for compliance is applied and compliance increases and aberrant behaviors decrease" (p. 219).

In another experiment Parrish, Cataldo, Kolko, Neef, and Egel (1986) formally tested the hypothesis that compliance and inappropriate behaviors are inversely related. Not only did they reinforce compliance to observe the impact on disruptive behavior, they also punished and reinforced disruptive behavior to observe the impact on compliance. Subjects were 3 males and 1 female, ages ranging from 3 years and 1 month to 5 years and 3 months, who had moderate to mild mental retardation. Dependent measures included compliance, aggression, disruption, property destruction, and pica. When compliance was reinforced with praise, inappropriate behavior decreased. When inappropriate behaviors were met with verbal social disapproval (and hence reinforced), compliance decreased, and when a DRO contingency functioned to punish inappropriate behaviors, compliance improved.

A second follow-up to the Russo et al. (1981) investigation was conducted by Cataldo, Ward, Russo, Riordan, and Bennett (1986). Subjects were four children with a mean age of 5.5 and IQ scores ranging from dull normal to profoundly retarded. Once again, results demonstrated that compliance and at least one problem behavior covaried inversely for each subject. Of particular interest were data showing that not all inappropriate behavior covaried with compliance. For example, data from one boy revealed that instruction-following behavior increased during the reinforcement for compliance condition, but climbing behavior was not reduced. These data suggest that, in this particular case, the consequences that reinforced climbing were not the same as those that reinforced compliance. This detracts from the explanation that compliance and disruption are inversely related because of incompatible rates of occurrence or physical incompatibility. Rather, they are related with respect to their functional consequences—reinforcement.

The purpose of the basic research on response covariation is to demonstrate and analyze the inverse functional relations between compliance and some disruptive behaviors in analog settings. In response to these analog studies, subsequent research demonstrated the applicability of response covariation analyses in natural environments. For example, Mace, Kratochwill and Fiello (1983) presented a case study of a 19-year-old male who had severe mental retardation and resided in a state mental retardation facility. Dependent measures were tantrums, aggression, and compliance. Baseline revealed substantial rates of tantrums and aggression. Compliance training consisted of praise and positive physical contact contingent upon compliant responses. Physical guidance was used to prompt incorrect responses. Results of the treatment showed that tantrums and aggression decreased concurrent with compliance training, even though the disruptive behavior was not targeted in compliance training. Furthermore, the study demonstrated the applicability of the procedure across therapists, settings, and maintenance in an 8-month follow-up.

Synthesizing Analyses of Controlling Variables

Recent studies have synthesized elements of research on functional analysis and response covariation to demonstrate how a combination of these analytic frameworks is applicable to treating aggressive and disruptive behaviors. Slifer, Ivancic, Parrish, Page, and Burgio (1986) presented a case study with a 13-year-old male who had profound mental retardation. Dependent variables included aggression, compliance, destruction to self or property, pica, and loud and abrupt vocalizations. During a behavioral assessment, the child was observed in three conditions: a demand condition, where he was required to participate in educational activities; a social disapproval condition, where verbal reprimands were provided contingent upon undesired behaviors; and a play condition, where the child simply played. Results showed high rates of inappropriate behavior in the demand conditions, suggesting that the aggressive behavior was negatively reinforced by withdrawal of the demand. Treatment sessions consisted of food reinforcement and praise contingent upon compliance, manual guidance following noncompliance, and not allowing aggression to terminate demands but instead treating it as noncompliance and providing manual guidance. In effect, aggression was placed on extinction. Food reinforcement for compliance was faded from continuous, to a fixed ratio 2 schedule of reinforcement, to praise only. Data clearly showed that aggression decreased after treatment was initiated. In addition, the rates of destructive and disruptive behaviors also subsided during this treatment and the effect generalized to family members who conducted some of the treatment sessions. Performance remained improved over a 12-week follow-up.

Slifer et al. (1986) hypothesized five processes that contributed to the outcome. First, the presentation of reinforcers may have made the demand condition less aversive and thus less reinforcing from which to escape. Second, manually guiding noncompliant responses, despite aggression, served to extinguish the escape properties of aggression. Third, escape was extinguished, thereby increasing the strength of other behaviors. Fourth, compliance was incompatible with aggression and disruption. Fifth, noncompliance may have been an early component in a chain of responses leading up to aggression.

A study incorporating elements of both functional analysis and response covariation was conducted by Carr and Durand (1985a). Subjects were four children who had developmental delays, two males and two females, with an average age of 12 and an average PPVT mental age score of 4. The researchers performed an initial functional analysis to determine variables maintaining aggression, tantrums, self-injury, opposition, out of seat, and stripping. Two children were more disruptive in a condition where difficult tasks were presented. Results suggested that escape from the difficult task was the negative reinforcing event maintaining disruption, so the children were taught communicative responses such as "I don't understand," designed to prompt teachers to provide assistance and thereby making the task less demanding. Another child was disruptive when adult attention was sparse. This child was taught to solicit praise from the teacher with statements such as "Am I doing good work?" In each case, disruptive behaviors decreased in frequency after communication training. The authors hypothesized that disruptive behavior initially functioned as a communicative response. Training a more appropriate communicative response ameliorated the need for the inappropriate response (see Carr, 1985; Carr & Durand, 1985b, for a more thorough theoretical analysis). Also, an undesirable behavior was reduced even though it was not directly targeted for intervention.

Compared with DRO and punishment procedures (to be described), interventions that rely on functional analysis and increasing appropriate alternative responses that are functionally related to aggression and disruption have a number of advantages. Providing specific consequences for the occurrence/nonoccurrence of a specified behavior modifies one response at a time, whereas analyses of controlling variables can influence multiple target behaviors. Acceptable alternative responses are directly taught. Also, the potential for generalization and maintenance is greater because controlling variables are manipulated. Compared with punishment, this is an ethical alternative that the social community can readily accept. It also reduces the possibility of unwanted side effects sometimes seen in punishment programs (Azrin & Holz, 1966; Newsom, Favell, & Rincover, 1983; Risley, 1968).

Further research must isolate conditions or behaviors that are not amenable to improved rates of compliance. In addition, practical problems may evolve when, for example, aggressive children are taught appropriate escape responses from educational settings.

PUNISHMENT

Punishment techniques have been used successfully for a number of years as components of multielement programs designed to decrease the rate of aggressive and disruptive behaviors (Matson & DiLorenzo, 1984). A comprehensive analysis of punishment procedures is presented by O'Brien in this monograph. For our purposes we have described recent representative studies designed to eliminate aggressive and/or disruptive behavior.

Time-Out

Time-out is a procedure in which access to reinforcement is removed following the occurrence of an undesired target response. The removal of reinforcing events should serve as a punisher for the preceding behavior. Early research on time-out illustrated many successful variations, including isolating the individual in a room or a corner of a room, removing materials that provide reinforcement, and withdrawing social reinforcement.

Determining events that function as reinforcers is an essential precursor to successful time-out. For example, prior to restricting access to social interactions contingent upon disruptive behavior, it must be determined that social interactions will reinforce behavior. Otherwise, the use of time-out might function as a negative reinforcer for the target behavior by removing social situations contingent upon disruptive behavior. Solnick, Rincover, and Peterson (1977) demonstrated that the degree of response suppression is a function of the amount of pleasurable events normally available in the "time-in" milieu. The same study showed that time-out was more effective when autistic children were physically restrained from self-stimulating during the time-out intervals. These examples illustrate the subtleties of creating a reinforcing environment from which the client can be removed and assuring that the time-out setting is not reinforcing.

In response to suggestions that self-stimulation during time-out reduces the efficacy of time-out, Rolider and Van Houten (1985) described a movement suppression time-out designed to suppress self-stimulation during the time-out interval. Four separate experiments were conducted with six children who had developmental disabilities. Movement suppression consisted of time-out in a corner, chin against the corner, both hands behind the back, feet close together touching the wall. The children were pressed into the corner if they moved and firmly instructed to remain still. Data revealed that the procedure was superior to contingent restraint and traditional time-out in reducing self-injurious and aggressive behavior. Furthermore, data suggested that the degree of movement suppressed in time-out was positively correlated with the degree to which the disruptive behavior was suppressed, supporting the Solnick et al. (1977) contention that self-stimulation can overcome the otherwise punishing impact of time-out. Given the careful staff training required, the intensity of the movement suppression described, and the possible relevance of this procedure to the numerous individuals who emit self-stimulatory behavior, this technique deserves further inquiry.

Recent analyses of time-out have focused on whether to delay release from time-out when disruptive behavior is occurring and on creative ways to manage highly aggressive and disruptive behavior. A standard aspect of time-out is maintaining the client in time-out until disruptive acts have ceased (Bostow & Bailey, 1969; Hobbs & Forehand, 1975). In an evaluation of this, Mace, Page, Ivancic, and O'Brien (1986) compared two procedures to release clients from time-out: (a) delaying the release until 15 seconds had passed without objectionable behavior and (b) releasing the client regardless of the behavior emitted during time-out. Three children in an inpatient hospital for individuals with developmental disabilities served as subjects. An ABAC reversal design combined with a multiple baseline across conditions revealed that both procedures reduced aggressive/disruptive behaviors to near zero and that the rate of aberrant responses in time-out was comparable. The results are consistent with the standard time-out practice of delaying release until the inappropriate behavior has ceased, and therefore certainly warrant further research. Yet it was clear that time-out without contingent delay can be as effective as the procedure with delay under some circumstances.

A study examining how disruption during time-out influences its effectiveness was conducted by Luiselli and Greenidge (1982). A 12-year-old female who had severe retardation, was legally blind, and had a severe to profound hearing loss, received a 2-minute time-out for striking people. In the first treatment phase, the client consistently left a time-out chair and reentered the learning area. Aggression decreased mildly, but the classroom was disrupted. In treatment number two, the time-out area was located in a 6 foot by 4 foot room separated by a tumbling mat. The client dislodged the mat frequently and aggression increased. In a third condition, a small room was utilized for time-out and the door accessing the room was closed. After escape from time-out was eliminated, aggression ceased to occur over a 7-month follow-up. This illustrated how the suppressive effects of time-out are enhanced when the procedure is designed to overcome countercontrol.

A novel time-out procedure designed to reduce the violent aggression of a 23-year-old severely retarded and psychotic male was described by Foxx, Foxx, Jones, and Kiely (1980). Numerous attempts to control the client's aggression had failed. Time-out for aggression consisted of a 24-hour social isolation program. When the client was aggressive or destructive, he was restrained to prevent further damage and required to lie on his bed for 10 minutes. Then he was denied social contact for 24 hours, during which he wore a white hospital gown that indicated to staff not to interact with him socially. Toys and clothes were removed from his living quarters and people only spoke to him when necessary; otherwise they walked away. During the first few months the client was often violent during isolation. Twice he was in isolation for more than half a week. But the data show that over the course of months the violent, aggressive outbursts became less frequent and less intense, and emergency injections of Thorazine were dramatically reduced. The authors addressed ethical concerns by pointing out that the client was dangerous to himself and others, and that all less restrictive procedures had failed.

Aversive Techniques

In contrast to time-out, where access to reinforcement is removed, aversive procedures require that a noxious event be presented to a client contingent upon a display of undesired behavior. This is frequently described as *corporal punishment* by the lay public and *negative punishment* by behavior analysts.

Aversive punishing consequences are appropriate for programmatic effects designed to suppress behaviors that cause self-injury or pain, or permit increased mobility from restraint (Martin, 1975; Stolz et al., 1978). Such procedures should only be used after documented reinforcement programs have failed. Staff must be qualified professionals and concurrent shaping and reinforcement programs should focus on the acquisition of appropriate behavior.

Visual screening is a mild form of aversive punishment that is comparable to time-out in that it blocks access to reinforcement from visual sources, yet it is more severe because it requires contingent visual restriction. Early research on facial screening demonstrated applications to self-injurious and stereotypic behaviors (see Singh, 1981, for a review). More recently, facial screening has been demonstrated effective in reducing disruptive behaviors. Examples include reduced frequencies of spoon banging (Horton, 1987), public genital self-stimulation (Barmann & Murray, 1981), and loud screaming (Dick & Jackson, 1983).

A representative study by Singh, Winton, and Dawson (1982) illustrated the efficacy of this procedure. The targeted response was short loud screams. During treatment sessions, a bib was tied around the client's neck and whenever she screamed the bib was placed over her face without restricting breathing. The facial screen was removed after 1 minute without screaming or resistance to the bib. A multiple baseline design across three settings revealed immediate declines and eventual elimination of screaming following application of the facial screen. A 6-month follow-up revealed the rate of screaming to be less than twice per month.

Facial screening has a number of advantages. It is easy to use, cost effective, portable, easy to train staff and parents, and safe for the client. Therefore, it is ethically preferable to more aversive techniques.

Other punishment procedures recently found effective in suppressing disruptive/aggressive behaviors include aversive gustatory stimulation (Altmeyer, Williams, & Sams, 1985), contingent exercise (Luce, Delquadri, & Hall, 1980), ammonia spirits (Doke, Wolery, & Sumberg, 1983), and electric shock (Foxx, McMorrow, Bittle, & Bechtel, 1986). As an example of noxious tastes, Altmeyer et al. (1985) decreased aggressive biting incidents emitted by a 16-year-old blind female who had severe mental retardation by using contingent applications of Tabasco Sauce (sprayed into the girl's mouth) along with time-out and a DRO schedule.

Luce et al. (1980) used an ABAB design to analyze the effects of contingent exercise on aggressive hitting by a 7-year-old child who had developmental delay. Following each hit the boy was required to stand up and sit down on the floor 10 times. Initially, physical prompts were required, but these were withdrawn quickly. Hitting responses decreased rapidly and showed complete elimination during an 18-month follow-up. Advantages of contingent exercise noted by the authors were short punishment trials (lasting less than 30 seconds), less need for manual guidance, and a relatively subtle technique allowing application in many settings. However, one possible difficulty is the application of the technique with noncompliant children.

Doke et al. (1983) demonstrated how to use ammonia contingently in a case study with a 7-year-old autistic boy who had moderate mental retardation. Results showed that contingent application of ammonia spirits, ½ inch beneath the nostrils, produced an abrupt and dramatic decrease in the physical aggression and high-pitched inappropriate vocalizations.

Rarely has shock been used to treat aggressive behavior (Fehrenbach & Thelen, 1982), but it was recently applied (Foxx, McMorrow, Bittle, & Bechtel, 1986) in an attempt to control physical assaults and destructive behavior by a 20-year-old institutionalized male who had mild mental retardation. The history of intense violence, previous unsuccessful procedures, the dangerousness of this client's behavior to others, and the lack of an educational experience as a result of this behavior was used to justify shock as a treatment.

Subjective observation by the authors suggested that aggression was negatively reinforced by withdrawal of demands. In treatment, aggressive acts were followed by a 1-second shock delivered directly via a handheld stimulator and compliance was followed by vocal praise and physical affection, along with other positive reinforcement procedures. As compliance improved, the program was transferred to personnel on other units. Results showed that the intensity and rate of aggressive/destructive acts decreased substantially over the course of months. In addition, it was possible to discontinue psychotropic medications. The authors emphasized that the combination of two components played a significant role in the client's improvement—shock for aggression and an extinction of escape/avoidance.

Explicit in all punishment research is the necessity of a positive reinforcement component. This is not simply an ethical consideration; rather, both basic and applied behavior analysis research shows that punished responses will likely be replaced by other behaviors that serve the same function. Therefore, it is possible that another inappropriate behavior may replace the punished response if an appropriate behavior is not targeted for increase. In practice this means that staff should reinforce appropriate adaptive skills.

As in almost all areas of applied behavior analysis, further research would add to the technology of punishment. For example, time-out without contingent delay was found effective (Mace et al., 1986) and the parameters responsible for this need investigation. Social isolation time-out resembles the natural consequences of aggression and merits more detailed analysis. Visual screening is the least intrusive of the corporal punishments reviewed, yet it was quite effective. A number of the punishment techniques require

great staff effort. Foxx and Livesay (1984) suggested that effortful procedures are more likely to be discontinued after the researchers leave the
applied setting. The social validity of these procedures would be greatly
enhanced if it could be shown that effective techniques are used following
the experimenters' departure.

COMPARATIVE EFFICACY

Following the presentation of a host of effective techniques that suppress and/or replace aggressive and disruptive behavior, it is tempting to
compare the efficacy of the procedures. However, it is imperative that we
avoid simplistic comparisons of one technique versus another lest we arrive
at a decision before the data are complete. That is, before making comparisons it must be clear that the technology presented represents the most
effective use of the procedures. Otherwise, the resulting comparison might
hinder further research on the procedures found to have the least impact.
Thus, research should focus on isolating parameters that contribute to and
detract from each technique (Van Houten, 1987).

After such parametric investigations are conducted, it may even be
clearer that straightforward comparisons are difficult. First, most effective
treatment programs use more than one procedure. Even more important,
so many variables contribute to effective elimination and replacement of
aggression and disruption that there probably is no "best" way. Given the
complex clients involved in aggression and disruption, it is likely that
between-subject comparisons will be inappropriate. Even within-subject
comparisons of one procedure are unlikely to provide satisfactory information because generalization across individuals is never guaranteed. The
reason for questioning the likelihood of generalization across subjects was
made clear in the research attempting to isolate controlling variables, where
analysis indicated that the variables maintaining similar responses can never
be assumed to be the same (Carr & Durand, 1985a).

The "best" technique is, therefore, an individual functional analysis of
the variables that control each client's behavior; and, for each client, an
analysis for each undesired response is necessary. For example, Carr and
Durand (1985a) showed that the aggressive/disruptive behavior of two subjects was negatively reinforced by withdrawal of a demand, for a third
subject it was maintained by attention, and for a fourth subject it was
maintained by a combination of the two. Cataldo et al. (1986) revealed that
compliance covaried with many aggressive/disruptive behaviors of a child,
but not with all of them. The time-out research emphasized the necessity
of assuring that removal from pleasant events could in fact function to

reinforce a subject's behavior. Following assessment, selection of effective procedures can be based on client, setting, and staff characteristics.

Such a conclusion brings us back to the basic characteristic of all good behavior therapy: good assessment. Research that focused on isolating controlling variables received minimal attention before 1980, but is currently receiving greater attention. It is encouraging to note its growth. Research on parameters influencing the efficacy of isolated procedures should continue, but until research on controlling variables realizes equal stature, those procedures will never be maximally effective.

REFERENCES

Altmeyer, B. K., Williams, D. E., & Sams, V. (1985). Treatment of severe self-injurious and aggressive biting. *Journal of Behaviour Therapy and Experimental Psychiatry, 16*, 169–172.

Azrin, N. H., Hake, D. F., Holz, W. C., & Hutchinson, R. R. (1965). Motivational aspects of escape from punishment. *Journal of the Experimental Analysis of Behavior, 8*, 31–44.

Azrin, N. H., & Holz, W. C. (1966). Punishment. In W. K. Honig (Ed.), *Operant behavior: Areas of research and application* (pp. 380–447). New York: Appleton-Century-Crofts.

Barmann, B. C., & Murray, W. J. (1981). Suppression of inappropriate sexual behavior by facial screening. *Behavior Therapy, 12*, 730–735.

Barton, L. E., Brulle, A. R., & Repp, A. C. (1986). Maintenance of therapeutic change by momentary DRO. *Journal of Applied Behavior Analysis, 19*, 277–282.

Bates, P., & Wehman, P. (1977). Behavior management with the mentally retarded: An empirical analysis of the research. *Mental Retardation, 42*, 9–12.

Billingsley, F. F., & Neel, R. S. (1985). Competing behaviors and their effects on skill generalization and maintenance. *Analysis and Intervention in Developmental Disabilities, 5*, 357–372.

Bostow, D. E., & Bailey, J. B. (1969). Modification of severe disruptive and aggressive behavior using brief time-out and reinforcement procedures. *Journal of Applied Behavior Analysis, 2*, 31–37.

Carr, E. G. (1985). Behavioral approaches to language and communication. In E. Schopler & G. Mesilov (Eds.), *Current issues in autism: Volume 3, Communication problems in autism* (pp. 37–57). New York: Plenum.

Carr, E. G., & Durand, V. M. (1985a). Reducing behavior problems through functional communication training. *Journal of Applied Behavior Analysis, 18*, 111–126.

Carr, E. G., & Durand, V. M. (1985b). The social communicative basis of severe behavior problems in children. In S. Reiss & R. Bootzin (Eds.), *Theoretical issues in behavior therapy* (pp. 219–254). New York: Academic Press.

Carr, E. G., & Newsom, C. (1985). Demand-related tantrums: Conceptualization and treatment. *Behavior Modification, 9*, 403–426.

Carr, E. G , Newsom, C. D., & Binkoff, J. A. (1980). Escape as a factor in the aggressive behavior of two retarded children. *Journal of Applied Behavior Analysis, 13*, 101–117.

Cataldo, M. F., Ward, E. M., Russo, D. C., Riordan, M., & Bennett, C. (1986). Compliance and correlated problem behavior in children: Effects of contingent and noncontingent reinforcement. *Analysis and Intervention in Development Disabilities, 6*, 265–282.

Cipani, E. (1981). Modifying food spillage behavior in an institutionalized retarded client. *Journal of Behaviour Therapy and Experimental Psychiatry, 12*, 261–265.

Dick, D. M., & Jackson, H. J. (1983). The reduction of stereotypic screaming in a severely retarded boy through a visual screening procedure. *Journal of Behaviour Therapy and Experimental Psychiatry, 14*, 363–367.

Doke, L., Wolery, M., & Sumberg, C. (1983). Treating chronic aggression. Effects and side effects of response-contingent ammonia spirits. *Behavior Modification, 7*, 531–556.

Fehrenbach, P. A., & Thelan, M. H. (1982). Behavioral approaches to the treatment of aggression. *Behavior Modification, 6,* 465–497.

Foxx, C. L., Foxx, R. M., Jones, J. R., & Kiely, D. (1980). Twenty-four hour social isolation. A program for reducing the aggressive behavior of a psychotic-like retarded adult. *Behavior Modification, 4,* 130–144.

Foxx, R. M., & Livesay, J. (1984). Maintenance of response suppression following overcorrection: A 10-year retrospective examination of eight cases. *Analysis and Intervention of Developmental Disabilities, 4,* 65–79.

Foxx, R. M., McMorrow, M. J., Bittle, R. G., & Bechtel, D. R. (1986). The successful treatment of a dually-diagnosed deaf man's aggression with a program that included contingent electric shock. *Behavior Therapy, 17,* 170–186.

Foxx, R. M., McMorrow, M. J., Fenlon, S., & Bittle, R. G. (1986). The reductive effects of reinforcement procedures on the genital stimulation and stereotypy of a mentally retarded adolescent male. *Analysis and Intervention in Developmental Disabilities, 6,* 239–248.

Friman, P. C., Barnard, J. D., Altman, K., & Wolf, M. M. (1986). Parent and teacher use of DRO and DRI to reduce aggressive behavior. *Analysis and Intervention in Developmental Disabilities, 6,* 319–330.

Hayes, S. C., Nelson, R. O., & Jarrett, R. B. (1987). The treatment utility of assessment: A functional approach to evaluating assessment quality. *American Psychologist, 42,* 963–974.

Hobbs, S. A., & Forehand, R. (1975). Effects of differential release from time-out on children's deviant behavior. *Journal of Behaviour Therapy and Experimental Psychiatry, 6,* 256–257.

Homer, A. L., & Peterson, L. (1980). Differential reinforcement of other behavior: A preferred response elimination procedure. *Behavior Therapy, 11,* 449–471.

Horton, S. V. (1987). Reduction of disruptive mealtime behavior by facial screening. A case study of a mentally retarded girl with long-term follow-up. *Behavior Modification, 11,* 53–64.

Luce, S. C., Delquadri, J., & Hall, R. V. (1980). Contingent exercise: A mild but powerful procedure for suppressing inappropriate verbal and aggressive behavior. *Journal of Applied Behavior Analysis, 13,* 583–594.

Luiselli, J. K. (1984). Treatment of an assaultive, sensory-impaired adolescent through a multicomponent behavioral program. *Journal of Behaviour Therapy and Experimental Psychiatry, 15,* 71–78.

Luiselli, J. K., & Greenidge, A. (1982). Behavioral treatment of high-rate aggression in a rubella child. *Journal of Behaviour Therapy and Experimental Psychiatry, 13,* 152–157.

Luiselli, J. K., & Slocumb, P. R. (1983). Management of multiple aggressive behaviors by differential reinforcement. *Journal of Behaviour Therapy and Experimental Psychiatry, 14,* 343–347.

Mace, F. C., Kratochwill, T. R., & Fiello, R. A. (1983). Positive treatment of aggressive behavior in a mentally retarded adult. *Behavior Therapy, 14,* 689–696.

Mace, F. C., Page, T. J., Ivancic, M. T., & O'Brien, S. (1986). Effectiveness of brief time-out with and without contingent delay: A comparative analysis. *Journal of Applied Behavior Analysis, 19,* 79–86.

Marchetti, A. G. (1987). Wyatt v. Stickney: A consent decree. *Research in Developmental Disabilities, 8,* 249–259.

Martin, R. (1975). *Legal challenges to behavior modification: Trends in schools, corrections, and mental health.* Champaign, IL: Research Press.

Matson, J. L., & DiLorenzo, T. M. (1984). *Punishment and its alternatives.* New York: Springer.

Newsom, C. Favell, J. G., & Rincover, A. (1983). The side effects of punishment. In S. Axelrod & J. Apsche (Eds.), *The effects of punishment on human behavior* (pp. 285–316). New York: Academic.

Nirje, B. (1969). The normalization principle and its human management implications. In R. Kugel & W. Wolfensberger (Eds.), *Changing patterns in residential services for the mentally retarded.* Washington, DC: President's Committee on Mental Retardation.

Parrish, J. M., Cataldo, M. F., Kolko, D. J., Neef, N. A., & Egel, A. L. (1986). Experimental analysis of response covariation among compliant and inappropriate behaviors. *Journal of Applied Behavior Analysis, 19,* 241–254.

Poling, A., & Ryan, C. (1982). Differential reinforcement of other behavior schedules: Therapeutic applications. *Behavior Modification, 6,* 3–21.

Polvinale, R. A., & Lutzker, J. R. (1980). Elimination of assaultive and inappropriate sexual behavior by reinforcement and social restitution. *Mental Retardation, 18,* 27–30.

Repp, A. C., Barton, L. E., & Brulle, A. R. (1983). A comparison of two procedures for programming the differential reinforcement of other behaviors. *Journal of Applied Behavior Analysis, 16,* 435–445.

Repp, A. C., & Brulle, A. R. (1981). Reducing aggressive behavior of mentally retarded persons. In J. L. Matson & J. R. McCartney (Eds.), *Handbook of behavior modification with the mentally retarded* (pp. 117–210). New York: Plenum Press.

Reynolds, G. S. (1961). Behavioral contrast. *Journal of the Experimental Analysis of Behavior, 4,* 57–71.

Risley, T. R. (1968). The effects and side-effects of punishing the autistic behaviors of a deviant child. *Journal of Applied Behavior Analysis, 1,* 21–34.

Rolider, A., & Van Houten, R. (1985). Movement suppression time-out for undesirable behavior in psychotic and severely developmentally delayed children. *Journal of Applied Behavior Analysis, 18,* 275–288.

Russo, D. C., Cataldo, M. F., & Cushing, P. J. (1981). Compliance training and behavioral covariation in the treatment of multiple behavior problems. *Journal of Applied Behavior Analysis, 14,* 209–222.

Singh, N. N. (1981). Current trends in the treatment of self-injurious behavior. In L. A. Barness (Ed.), *Advances in pediatrics* (Vol. 28). Chicago: Year Book Medical Publishers.

Singh, N. H., Winton, A. S., Dawson, M. J. (1982). Suppression of antisocial behavior by facial screening using multiple baseline and alternating treatment designs. *Behavior Therapy, 13,* 511–520.

Slifer, K. J., Ivancic, M. T., Parrish, J. M., Page, T. J., & Burgio, L. D. (1986). Assessment and treatment of multiple behavior problems exhibited by a profoundly retarded adolescent. *Journal of Behaviour Therapy and Experimental Psychiatry, 17,* 203–213.

Solnick, J. V., Rincover, A., & Peterson, C. R. (1977). Some determinants of the reinforcing and the punishing effects of time-out. *Journal of Applied Behavior Analysis, 10,* 415–424.

Stolz, S. B., & Associates. (1978). *Ethical issues in behavior modification.* San Francisco: Jossey-Bass.

Sulzer-Azaroff, B., & Mayer, G. R. (1977). *Applying behavior analysis procedures with children and youth.* New York: Holt, Rinehart, & Winston.

Van Houten, R. (1987). Comparing treatment techniques: A cautionary note. *Journal of Applied Behavior Analysis, 20,* 109–110.

Wolfensberger, W. (1972). *The principle of normalization in human services.* Toronto: National Institute on Mental Retardation.

Community-Referenced Research on Self-Stimulation

Robert L. Koegel
and
Lynn Kern Koegel
University of California, Santa Barbara

It is not uncommon to see children who have autism or other severe handicaps incessantly rocking back and forth, repetitiously moving their fingers in front of their eyes or flapping their hands in the air. These are just a few of the many thousands of self-stimulatory behaviors (also called *disturbances in motility, autistic mannerisms, autistic behavior, stereotyped behavior, stereotypic behavior,* or *stereotypies*) that may consume the majority of these children's waking hours (Repp & Barton, 1980). Some behaviors, such as those just mentioned, are quite obvious. Others can be more subtle, such as hyperventilating, manipulating the tongue inside of the mouth, or staring into space. The pervasiveness and negative social and educational impact of such behaviors has stimulated a considerable amount of clinical research attempts to treat self-stimulatory behavior.

However, in spite of massive efforts in many areas, this type of behavior has been very resistant to change and little practical benefit has been attained. The reason for this difficulty may lie in the fact that self-stimulatory behavior seems to represent response classes with controlling variables that are more difficult to assess and to manipulate than are those affecting many other behaviors. The purpose of this chapter, therefore, is twofold: to discuss research that helps to understand the relationship of controlling variables to self-stimulatory behavior; and, as a result of the above, to discuss productive avenues for community-referenced, nonaversive treatment research and development, with the potential for producing major social and educational benefits for children who have severe handicaps. This article is divided into three sections: a presentation of background material; a discussion of traditional avenues of treatment and their limita-

Acknowledgment. Preparation of this manuscript was supported in part by U.S. Department of Education, Special Education Program Research Contract No. 300-82-0362; by National Institute on Disability and Rehabilitation Research Cooperative Agreement No. G0087C0234; and by U.S. Public Health Service Research Grants MH28210 and MH39434 from the National Institute of Mental Health.

129

tions; and a discussion of how the early work has led to new approaches that are nonaversive, easily applicable in the community, and quite effective.

BACKGROUND

Treatment for self-stimulatory behaviors has proven to be a major concern in relation to several issues. First, such stereotyped behavior can stigmatize persons who have severe handicaps and may inhibit efforts to integrate such individuals into nonsegregated environments (Durand & Carr, 1987). Although not all types of self-stimulatory behavior are problematic (Dunlap, Dyer, & Koegel, 1983), researchers have indicated that children who have very severe handicaps and autism and who have certain types of self-stimulatory behavior are not likely to make substantial improvements (Rutter, 1966) or to learn even relatively simple new tasks under normal learning conditions (Koegel & Covert, 1972; Lovaas, Freitag, Kinder, Rubenstein, Schaeffer, & Simmons, 1966; Risley, 1968). For example, Lovaas, Litrownik, and Mann (1971) demonstrated that mute autistic children had seriously increased response latencies or did not respond at all to training stimuli while they were engaging in self-stimulatory behavior. This failure to respond was even more dramatically demonstrated by L. Silverman (personal communication, 1972), who showed that the effect was present even with very intense stimuli. That is, when she presented a high amplitude and sudden onset stimulus (a 110 dB blank fired from a starting pistol), nearby children who were engaged in self-stimulatory behavior showed no response either behaviorally or physiologically, as measured by videotapes and by galvanic skin response tests. Another study further supporting the severity of the problem was conducted by Koegel and Covert (1972) who showed that children who had autism did not learn a simple discrimination while engaged in self-stimulation. Additionally, other studies have shown that self-stimulatory behavior interferes with appropriate social behavior (Risley, 1968) and appropriate play (Koegel, Firestone, Kramme, & Dunlap, 1974).

In contrast, when self-stimulatory behavior is suppressed, one can observe dramatic improvements in the children's appropriate behaviors. The children not only demonstrate shorter response latencies but begin to respond where there was previously no response of any type (Lovaas et al., 1971). Further, correct responding increases under such conditions and has led to eventual learning of tasks that were not acquired while the children were previously engaged in self-stimulation. In addition, studies have reported increases in appropriate play (Koegel et al., 1974) and other types of socially desirable behavior (Risley, 1968). This inverse relationship between self-stimulation and appropriate responding is evident not only when self-stimulatory behavior is manipulated by external consequences, but also when it is naturally occurring at high or low levels (Koegel & Covert, 1972; Lovaas et al., 1971). Thus, as a whole, the literature shows that self-stimulatory behavior seems to be incompatible with the occurrence or establishment of many appropriate behaviors.

This leads to the very interesting question of why many children spend literally all day, every day, engaged in a behavior with virtually no social value or other apparent external benefit. The answer may lie in the fact that self-stimulation seems to provide reinforcing sensory input for such children (Lovaas et al., 1971; Lovaas, Newsom, & Hickman, 1987). This input can be obtained in a number of ways. For example, auditory input can be obtained by spinning an object on a hard surface and listening to its vibration. Likewise, poking and scratching body parts can provide tactile input, smelling objects can result in olfactory input, and finger manipulations in front of the eyes can provide visual and/or proprioceptive input.

From a theoretical point of view, it is possible that such sensory input may function as a competing reinforcer with other types of input that the environment provides (Dyer, 1987). This hypothesis is strengthened by data from Lovaas et al. (1971), who externally manipulated the children's self-stimulatory behavior. When the experimenter induced self-stimulatory behavior by providing external visual sensory input, the children demonstrated the same response latencies that occurred with the children's spontaneous self-stimulation. In an attempt to account for this incompatibility, Lovaas et al. (1971) postulated that (a) the reinforcing stimuli that are generated by self-stimulatory behavior are exclusive, and cannot, so to speak, be "enjoyed" during concurrent other stimulation; and (b) in children who have autism, the reinforcing stimuli that maintain social and intellectual behavior are so weak relative to self-stimulatory reinforcers as to leave a preponderance of self-stimulatory behavior (also see Dyer, 1987).

Regardless of the reason for self-stimulatory behavior, if any progress is to occur in the treatment and community integration of children who have autism, it seems crucial that this behavior be remediated. Unfortunately, self-stimulatory behavior has been very resistant to treatment. From a behavioral point of view, because the response (the self-stimulatory behavior) and the postulated reinforcer (the sensory input) are both controlled largely by the child, it may be very difficult to break the chain. In contrast, most other responses that are emitted by a child are or can be consequated by the environment. For example, consequences such as adult attention, which appear important for behaviors other than self-stimulation, are quite easy to manipulate.

However, much progress has been made and very promising avenues of research have been established. The remainder of this chapter will provide an overview and discussion of both traditional treatment approaches and a number of very promising, new community-referenced, nonaversive approaches that are emerging through steadily advancing lines of research.

TRADITIONAL APPROACHES
AND LIMITATIONS

Traditional treatment techniques can be categorized loosely into three areas as follows: extinction, time-out, and response-contingent aversive stimulation. These techniques have been investigated for many years and have varied in successfulness. However, they provide a foundation from which several innovative new community-based, nonaversive approaches directly follow.

Extinction

As a treatment technique, extinction involves withholding reinforcers known to maintain responding. For example, the most common type of extinction is ignoring the inappropriate behavior. Extinction may be desirable with a very small number of socially maintained repetitive behaviors, such as certain subtypes of delayed echolalia (Lovaas, Varni, Koegel, & Lorsch, 1977). However, in general, these techniques have been shown to be ineffective in reducing most self-stimulatory behavior (Newsom, Carr, & Lovaas, 1977; Rincover, Newsom, Lovass, & Koegel, 1977). It is logical that extinction would not be effective because, as discussed earlier, the response and reinforcing consequences seem to be controlled directly by the child; thus, with typical extinction procedures, there is no disruption of the consequence (i.e., possible sensory reinforcement). In addition, because the therapist typically does not interact with the child during traditional extinction procedures, such approaches might even provide increased opportunity for self-stimulation and may therefore result in sensory reinforcers for the inappropriate behavior (Solnick, Rincover, & Peterson, 1977).

Time-out

The success of time-out as a treatment technique for self-stimulatory behavior has been limited for reasons similar to those for extinction. The primary limitations of time-out relate to the fact that the relative reinforcing properties of the time-out versus the time-in environment are often in the wrong proportions. That is, with typical time-out procedures used to treat self-stimulation, the time-out environment may become more reinforcing than the time-in environment. For example, Solnik et al. (1977) unexpectedly discovered such problems when they tried to use time-out to reduce the frequency of tantrums in a 6-year-old girl who had autism. Unexpectedly, a subsequent increase in tantrums resulted. Further analysis utilizing a repeated reversal design indicated that the opportunity to engage in self-stimulatory behavior during the time-out period was apparently functioning as a very powerful reinforcer and causing an increase in her tantrums.

The above research suggests that teachers and parents using time-out monitor the child's behavior during time-out periods to determine whether the child engages in preferred behavior. If behaviors occur that can be reinforcing, time-out as a treatment may have unexpected and undesirable effects. In a second experiment detailed in the same article, the authors also showed that time-out can have both reinforcing and punishing effects, depending on the characteristics of the time-in environment. They utilized time-out with a 16-year-old youth who had severe retardation. When his time-in environment was enriched with new toys and social interaction, time-out functioned as a punisher. However, in an impoverished time-in setting that provided few toys and little social interaction, the same time-out procedure was ineffective.

Another area that remains relatively undocumented in the literature relates to the fact that time-out can be implemented in a number of different ways. That is, removal of the availability of reinforcement can be accomplished by removing materials the child is engaged in, removal of adult attention, exclusion of an ongoing activity or group without isolation, and exclusion of an ongoing activity or group with isolation. There have been suggestions that various types of time-out may function differently (Pendergrass, 1972; Sachs, 1973). The relative effectiveness of these procedures still warrants further research. However, the literature suggests that, as of now, time-out as a treatment for self-stimulatory behavior does not seem to be a technique of choice.

Response-Contingent Aversive Stimulation

Although much of the following research was done many years ago, and does not always have the number of dependent variables that we like to see today, the literature suggests that noxious stimuli presented contingently following self-stimulation have been consistent in at least temporarily showing rapid and dramatic increases in self-stimulation. For example, a verbal "no" paired with a brisk light slap on the hands has rapidly decreased self-stimulatory behavior in autistic children. Additionally, under such conditions, an inverse relationship with learning has been noted, with eventual acquisition of new tasks during these procedures (Koegel & Covert, 1972).

Similarly, reductions of autistic rocking were demonstrated following the command "no" and the vigorous shaking of a 6-year-old girl diagnosed as having diffuse brain damage (Risley, 1968). Finally, electric shock has been used in more severe cases of children who have not responded favorably to other techniques (Risley, 1968).

In an excellent review of 89 research studies related to the treatment of stereotypic responding, LaGrow and Repp (1984) determined that electric shock was the most effective single intervention procedure in terms of the mean rate of change for each intervention. However, in spite of its success, the use of electric shock and other painful procedures has been questioned on ethical grounds (Hobbs & Goswick, 1977, as cited in LaGrow & Repp, 1984). That is, such types of severe punishers raise a complex set of issues relating to defining, distinguishing, and proving that a procedure is effective versus "abusive" or "degrading." In an eloquent editorial of treatment abuse and its reduction, Schopler (1986) discussed the fact that, when parents cannot control their child's severely disruptive behavior, when there is no appropriate community support to contain or decrease their stress, and when the integrity of the family is seriously threatened, they may be vulnerable to even the most unsubstantiated claims for cure or relief. Unfortunately, such desperate parents often see extremely aversive therapy as their only hope, and the potential for abuse is great. Thus, in spite of their tremendous potential for effectiveness if utilized correctly, aversive stimulation techniques have remained controversial and relatively rarely used over the year.

However, some of the dramatic control over self-stimulatory behavior and its simultaneous inverse relationship with appropriate behaviors has led to alternative community-referenced technologies that have focused on the fact that dramatic increases in appropriate behaviors can be seen when self-stimulatory behavior is suppressed. These techniques are now being widely researched, and it is hoped that in the near future families will have support and professional personnel will be trained to teach both children and their parents how to deal successfully with severely disruptive behavior in a manner that will provide effective results while maintaining the respect and dignity of the severely handicapped individuals in the community. The following sections discuss such techniques.

NONAVERSIVE PROCEDURES

Nonaversive procedures dealing with self-stimulatory behavior will be categorized as *nonaversive response consequences* and *nonaversive antecedent procedures*. Both research avenues are based heavily on the findings in the above literature that show that appropriate behaviors have consistently covaried inversely when self-stimulatory behaviors are altered (Koegel et al., 1974). Therefore, researchers now have attempted to alter self-stimulatory behavior indirectly by treating appropriate behaviors that may inversely covary with self-stimulation.

Nonaversive Response Consequences

This category provided a promising starting point for nonaversive interventions and bridged the gap between the earlier more punitive interventions and the more completely nonaversive interventions discussed later in this article. This initial category is based heavily on positive reinforcement, but also relies somewhat on initial interruption of the self-stimulatory behavior through mild verbal reprimands, mild overcorrection, and/or mild physical restraint. With these last three categories, it is important to remember that they can and should be carried out very briefly in combination with other techniques and should be used nonaversively. However, like any procedure, the techniques can be abused and, because the latter two involve some physical contact between the clinician and child, could potentially be used incorrectly and cause discomfort to the child. Thus, following each section guidelines for the appropriate administration of the procedures will be discussed.

Positive Reinforcement

The two most commonly discussed types of positive reinforcement involve differential reinforcement of other behaviors (DRO) and differential reinforcement of incompatable behaviors (DRI) (LaVigna & Donnellan, 1986). Procedurally, DRO consists of reinforcing specified intervals of time that do not contain a particular inappropriate response. Schedules of DRO must consider initial DRO intervals so that they are small enough to provide success. Then gradual and systematic lengthening of the interval follows. An example of effective DRO programming was published by Repp, Deitz, and Deitz (1976). They reduced mentally retarded children's inappropriate behaviors such as hairtwirling, handbiting, and thumbsucking in individual settings and "talkouts" (i.e., speaking without permission, screaming, singing, whistling, or loud coughing) in a classroom setting. Initial DRO intervals for three retarded children in the individual settings ranged from 1 second to 1 minute and were then gradually increased to 5 minutes. In the classroom setting, children who had mild retardation were delivered mediating reinforcers (1 point) after 3-minute intervals. Ten accumulated points could be exchanged for either free time or ice cream. In both settings, the data demonstrated dramatic and substantial decreases repeatedly in both multiple baseline and reversal experimental designs. The authors suggested that the successfulness of their program may relate to carefully choosing initial time intervals (i.e., the mean interval between responses during baseline) and the use of individually selected reinforcers that had previously been shown to be effective for each subject.

DRI consists of contingently reinforcing behaviors that are incompatable with self-stimulation. For example, Favell (1973) utilized a multiple baseline design with three children who had severe and profound retardation and who had been observed to exhibit high rates of stereotypies. The participants were trained and reinforced for appropriate toy play (note that this is a nonaversive inverse application of the same variables described by Koegel et al., 1974). All three subjects, who previously had been uninterested in playing with toys, showed dramatic decreases in stereotypies while they were being trained and reinforced for appropriate toy play. Unfortunately, once the reinforcement was discontinued, no maintenance occurred and the children showed the same high pretreatment levels of stereotypies (see also Koegel et al., 1974). Favell (1973) suggested that, as the child eventually receives more natural reinforcers emanating from the toys themselves, more durable decreases in stereotypies may result.

The above findings raise an interesting question. That is, if the results are not durable, then just how effective are positive reinforcement procedures when used alone? Foxx and Azrin (1973) compared DRO with the use of overcorrection with other techniques and found DRO used alone to be the least effective method of reducing self-stimulation in two children who had severe retardation. Thus, positive reinforcement procedures used alone may not be as effective or rapid as other response inhibitory techniques. One reason for such limited effectiveness may be partly attributable to the fact that, if a child exhibits high levels of inappropriate behavior, opportunities to deliver reinforcers may be limited. One answer to such a situation may be to combine training of appropriate behavior with the simultaneous reinforcement of any attempts to respond (Koegel, O'Dell, & Dunlap, in press; Koegel, O'Dell, & Koegel, 1987) and other appropriate behavior emitted by the child during the training (Dunlap, 1984; Koegel & Koegel, 1986; Winterling, Dunlap, & O'Neill, 1987). Thus, the trainer would be teaching and reinforcing newly learned appropriate behaviors that the child was not previously emitting.

One must also be careful not to inadvertently reinforce an undesirable behavior. This frequently occurs in a situation where a child is reinforced after a prespecified time period. To overcome this problem, the clinician must be careful to deliver reinforcement only after a specific time period of no inappropriate behavior, regardless of how well the child is behaving at the end of the prespecified time interval (Dunlap, Koegel, Johnson, & O'Neill, 1987). Additionally, pure administration of positive reinforcement may result in satiation on the child's part. Thus, if reinforcers such as food are being used, they may not be as effective if they are being frequently administered, and it may be advantageous to try to incorporate a token or other secondary reward system as early as possible.

Finally, using only positive reinforcement procedures may be very time consuming and require constant vigilance on the part of the trainer. Therefore, while such procedures may be suitable or even desirable in an individual setting, they may also be difficult to implement when numerous children must be considered (Favell, 1973). Thus, while it is desirable to use positive reinforcement to build appropriate responses into a child's repertoire, a more rapid and effective program may result if positive reinforcement is used in combination with other techniques that will be discussed below.

Mild Reprimands/Verbal Commands

As a result of studies such as those discussed above showing that positive reinforcement procedures can result in covarying decreases in self-stimulatory behaviors, renewed interest has occurred in the use of more normalized verbal instructions, such as those that are typically used with nonhandicapped children. That is, it now should be possible to rely on much less aversive (and more socially acceptable) negative verbal consequences than has been possible in the past.

As a whole in the past, successful mild verbal reprimands or verbal commands such as "no" delivered contingently upon a response have typically been delivered just prior to the application of another more aversive procedure (Martin, Weller, & Matson, 1977), especially with children who have autism (Koegel & Covert 1972; Koegel et al., 1974; Risley, 1968). However, studies that have relied on auditory stimulation as a unitary procedure to treat stereotypic behavior have shown mixed results. For example, on the positive side Baumeister and Forehand (1972) gave the verbal command "stop rocking" contingent upon bodyrocking in three institutionalized adult males who were neither testable or verbal. This verbal reprimand resulted in decreases in bodyrocking to near zero levels. This was demonstrated in an ABAB design for 12 days with 15-minute sessions daily. Another study showed similar positive results, although Greene, Hoats, and Hornick (1970) used a different type of auditory stimulus (music distortion rather than a reprimand or command): Greene et al. (1970) interrupted music that was reinforcing to an institutionalized, blind, severely retarded 15-year-old boy with distortion when he engaged in disruptive rocking. Following the presentation of the distortion, the rocking rate was rapidly decelerated in a repeated reversal design.

In contrast to the above studies, Sachs (1973) found that a verbal "no" presented contingently upon self-stimulatory behaviors resulted in increases in the rate and number of self-stimulatory behaviors. Thus, while "no" may be subjectively considered to be aversive, in this study it functioned, if anything, as a positive reinforcer. This anomoly may be discussed in relation to several issues. First, it must be remembered that punishers must be individually defined (Sachs, 1973). Second, sternly saying "no" may rely more on its startle effects as a response suppressor and not very much on aversiveness. While this may be functional for some children, children who have autism have been shown to lack startle responses while engaged in self-stimulatory behavior and often may not be affected by such a procedure. Finally, Doke and Epstein (1975) have shown that verbal threats contingent upon inappropriate behaviors are not effective without previous association with backup punishers following the threat. Thus, a number of complex variables seem to interact in relation to the effectiveness of verbal interventions.

Finally, in consideration of carrying out such procedures nonaversively, it is important to remember that untrained lay individuals often resort to severe reprimands, such as shouting, which may provide undesirable and/ or demeaning models for children and peers and also may be disruptive to other children's learning in a classroom setting. Thus, the typical lay individual may require training in the use of verbal reprimands so that such individuals will not resort to verbal interactions that are not only socially undesirable, but ineffective as well. The literature now suggests that this is not necessary and one should follow through with verbal commands in a mild and contingent manner and in combination with other procedures (also see discussions below).

Mild Overcorrection

Overcorrection has been researched and discussed extensively in the literature. It is designed to require the misbehaving individual to overcorrect the environmental effects of the inappropriate act and/or to practice correct forms of relevant behavior in situations where the misbehavior commonly occurs (Foxx & Bechtel, 1982). Note that this procedure has built into it the notion of increasing an incompatible appropriate behavior. Thus, as with all of the other effective combinations discussed above, a mild suppressant combined with an increased appropriate behavior has been shown to be most effective.

Overcorrection has repeatedly been shown to be successful in reducing self-stimulatory behaviors. However, like any procedure, it has the potential to be misused and thus be either extremely unpleasant or even painful. Thus, while applying this procedure, its developers and others have proposed that the following guidelines be incorporated: (a) all verbal contacts (instructions and otherwise) be carried out in a matter-of-fact, nondemeaning manner; (b) any physical contact be used as a gentle prompt only, and be removed as soon as the misbehaver attempts to perform the desired appropriate (or overcorrection) behavior; and (c) the compliance training be carried out only as long as necessary to be effective (e.g., less than 2 minutes).

Common components to all overcorrection programs include the use of nonaversive verbal reprimands following the inappropriate behavior; a period of time-out from positive reinforcement (including removal from possible sensory reinforcement provided by the self-stimulatory behavior); compliance training, in which noncompliance is decreased by the immediate application of guidance whenever an instruction is not followed; and negatively reinforcing appropriate behavior when the individual is released from the successful completion of the overcorrection act (Epstein, Doke, Sajwaj, Sorrell, & Rimmer, 1974). Thus, while it is not directly discussed in the previous literature, one can observe that teaching the child an appropriate way to obtain sensory stimulation may be a central component of this procedure. In the case of self-stimulatory behaviors, one might therefore deduce that effective overcorrection treatment should consist of minimizing the duration of the self-stimulation episode by immediate teacher interruption; preventing self-stimulatory behavior during the overcorrection; directly teaching outward directed activities by manual guidance and instructions; providing positive reinforcement for outward directed activities; and transferring the sensory consequences from the self-stimulation to appropriate forms of behavior.

Overcorrection has been researched extensively and numerous studies have been published demonstrating its effectiveness with self-stimulatory behavior. For example, Martin et al. (1977) eliminated object-transferring in a 27-year-old woman who had profound retardation by requiring her to hold her arms in three positions—hand above head, hands outstretched to sides, and hands held to sides. Each position was maintained for a 15-second period. In another study, Freeman, Moss, Somerset, and Ritvo (1977) suppressed thumbsucking in a 24-month-old boy who had autism by holding his hands down to his sides for 30 seconds following each occurrence of thumbsucking. Finally, Barrett and Shapiro (1980) reduced trichiotillomania in a 7½-year-old girl who had severe mental retardation by requiring her to brush her hair appropriately for a 2-minute period contingent upon each observed instance of the inappropriate behavior.

As with the other procedures discussed in this paper, several investigators have compared overcorrection with other procedures and their results have been varied. For example, Harris and Wolchik (1979) analyzed time-out, DRO, and overcorrection for the suppression of self-stimulatory behavior in four young boys with "autistic-like" behavior. Their data showed that overcorrection resulted in immediate and dramatic declines in self-stimulation for all four boys. In contrast, time-out produced only mild reductions, and DRO caused decreases in self-stimulation in one child, increases in another, and no changes in the remaining two. In another study comparing mild physical restraint and overcorrection, Shapiro, Barrett, and Ollendick (1980) found the two procedures equally effective in treating the stereotypic behavior of three girls who had mental retardation. Additional studies have found that DRO failed to reduce masturbation in an 8-year-old mentally retarded, behaviorally disturbed boy (Luiselli, Helfen, Pemberton, & Reisman, 1977), while DRO and overcorrection used together eliminated the behavior in a relatively short period of time. Also, wheelchair mobility as an overcorrection treatment contingent upon the occurrence of self-stimulatory behavior combined with social praise for appropriate toy play resulted in a reduction of self-stimulation, which DRO alone had failed to produce (see also Roberts, Iwata, McSween, & Desmond, 1979). Again, in practically every instance, one can observe that *the combination* of teaching an appropriate substitute behavior while interfering with, interrupting, or otherwise decelerating the self-stimulation has been most effective.

From a practical point of view, it is also important to consider the fact that, like many other treatment procedures, overcorrection may produce direct effects, but there is often lack of generalization across settings (Harris & Wolchik, 1979; Matson & Stephens, 1981). Teacher training (Coleman, Whitman, & Johnson, 1979) and/or parent training (Foxx & Azrin, 1973) of the procedure may be helpful in decreasing generalization problems somewhat, and maintenance problems may be overcome by systematic fading of the trainer (Matson & Stephens, 1981) and/or pairing a verbal warning with the procedure that can be utilized after the procedure is terminated (Barrett & Shapiro, 1980; Doke & Epstein, 1975). However, generalization questions still remain an important research area.

Finally, overcorrection procedures as discussed in the literature do not always consider time effectiveness. An overcorrection period such as 20 minutes (Foxx & Azrin, 1973) may often be too time-consuming to use in situations other than a one-on-one setting. However, briefer periods, such as 1 minute, may be just as effective, require a lesser investment of teacher time (Luiselli, Pemberton, & Helfen, 1978), and be less aversive for the child.

In summary, an overview of the numerous studies related to the use of overcorrection suggests that overcorrection may be effective in reducing self-stimulatory behavior, but even more effective from an educative point of view in relation to the covariation effect discussed by Koegel and Covert (1972) if used with other intervention techniques such as DRO and/or DRI. However, this procedure, like other techniques, has not been effective with all children. Thus, as with all techniques, careful analysis of both pre- and postimplementation is necessary. The major point being stressed here, however, is that the covarying aspect of self-stimulation and other more appropriate forms of obtaining sensory input may rest at the heart of the most effective interventions.

Mild Physical Restraint

Mild physical restraint consists of mildly and briefly (as opposed to using a straight jacket or soft or hard ties, etc.) immobilizing the part of the body involved in self-stimulation until the self-stimulation subsides. This procedure, like overcorrection, can be abused such that it can cause discomfort or pain to a person if used improperly. It is recommended that this procedure be used only as a prompt to remind the person who is engaged in self-stimulation not to do so, or to interfere with the self-stimulation long enough to prompt an appropriate behavior. Therefore, the prompt need only consist of very gentle and brief immobilization by the therapist.

Most studies utilizing mild physical restraint have either compared it with or used it in combination with other procedures. For example, Shapiro et al. (1980) found physical restraint and overcorrection to be equally effective when used alone, with only modest improvements in appropriate behaviors for both procedures used together. Their physical restraint procedure, used with three children who had mental retardation and who exhibited inappropriate stereotypic mouthing or face-patting behavior, consisted of a verbal warning (e.g., "No, Marcia, hands out of your mouth") and manually restraining the children's hands on the table for 30 seconds. In a later study comparing no treatment, physical restraint, and overcorrection in an alternating treatments design, Ollendick, Shapiro, and Barrett (1981) found differential subject effects. That is, while both treatments were better than no treatment, two of three mentally retarded, emotionally disturbed children showed greater decreases in stereotypic behavior when overcorrection was applied, and the other responded more favorably to physical restraint. Also, task performance gradually increased under all conditions, suggesting that none of the treatments in and of themselves had any differential educative value.

In contrast to the above results, utilizing physical restraint with DRO was found to produce immediate and substantial decreases in the stereotypic body contortions of a 9-year-old girl who had mental retardation (Barkley & Zupnick, 1976). Their procedure consisted of saying "no" to the child several times while grasping her hands and holding them firmly to her sides until the responding seemed to subside. The subsequent DRO consisted of delivering social praise and M&M candies following completion of successful time intervals without stereotypy. Thus, when one compares studies a consistent finding emerges, showing that mild suppression combined with teaching an alternative means of obtaining sensory input continues to be the most effective intervention.

Nonaversive Antecedent Procedures

The use of antecedent behavioral interventions is a relatively recent area of research as it relates to self-stimulatory behavior. However, these techniques, which can be seen to be directly evolved from the research discussed in all of the previous sections of this article, may hold the most promise of all for providing community-referenced nonaversive treatment. Several procedures involving the use of antecendent interventions include the use of task variation, functionally equivalent communicative alternatives, *a priori* specially assessing reinforcers, antecedent physical exercise programs, and sensory assessment and extinction.

At this point it is necessary to mention that drug therapy could also be considered an antecedent intervention. However, drug therapy is quite controversial both in terms of its lack of effectiveness in reducing self-stimulatory behavior in some patients (Berkson, 1965) and in producing variable results in others (Marholin, Touchette, & Stewart, 1979). Also, undesirable side effects, both immediate and long term, have been a concern of many (Yarbrough, Sentat, Perel, Webster, & Lombardi, 1987). Finally, our own research has been based on the use of behavioral procedures rather than on drug therapies. Thus, for all of the above reasons, the following sections will focus entirely on behavioral procedures and/or the interaction of behavioral and physiological variables.

Teaching and relying on antecedent procedures is a conceptually valuable treatment approach because it does not require the difficult task of breaking the stimulus-response-consequence chain, which in the case of self-stimulatory behavior may be controlled predominantly by the child (as discussed above). Additionally, antecedent interventions may function as preventative measures, thus eliminating the reliance on response consequences that can so easily be misused. The following sections discuss various antecedent procedures.

Task Variation

Winterling et al. (1987) have investigated the influence of task variation on the aberrant responding (including self-stimulatory behavior) of three individuals. Their experimental procedure consisted of comparing a constant task treatment condition and a varied task treatment condition. During the constant task condition, a single instructional task was presented repeatedly until the child learned the task or until the session ended. In the varied task condition, the same instructional task was presented; however, it was interspersed with four other discrimination tasks that had previously been acquired. Thus, the new task was not presented more than two consecutive times without presenting an already acquired task. These interspersed tasks were hypothesized to have two functions: a rehearsal function to improve durability of learning; and, more importantly, a motivating function by providing opportunities to reinforce task-directed work. Their results showed that such task interspersal repeatedly resulted in a reduction of aberrant responding. Furthermore, the average number of trials of criterion was much lower in the interspersal condition. Therefore, the authors seem to have provided a simple, nonpunitive strategy to decrease aberrant behavior and improve learning in individuals who have severe handicaps (see also Dunlap, 1984; Koegel & Koegel, 1986; Neef, Iwata, & Page, 1980).

Functionally Equivalent Communicative Alternatives

Durand and Carr (1987) assessed the influence of social variables on the stereotypic behavior of four children who had developmental disabilities. They found in their first experiment that the childrens' self-stimulation (i.e., bodyrocking and handflapping) was unaffected by reduced rates of adult attention. However, whenever task difficulty was increased, self-stimulatory behavior also increased. These data suggest that some of the variables maintaining self-stimulatory behavior may involve escape from task demands. In a second experiment, the authors further tested this hypothesis by removing task materials for a 10-second period contingent on self-stimulatory behavior. Their results showed that the time-out was associated with increased rates of stereotyped responding. The children engaged in high rates of stereotypic behavior during work periods and low rates when task demands were removed. These findings support the results of their first experiment, demonstrating that the self-stimulatory behaviors were functioning as an escape from task demands. With these results in mind, the experimenters developed an intervention for the self-stimulatory behavior in which each student was taught to say "Help me" following an incorrect task-related response. As a function of the communicative treatment, substantial reductions in bodyrocking and handflapping were recorded. Thus, this suggests that the communicative responses served the same function as the self-stimulatory behavior: to reduce the aversiveness of the demand. An important point to be emphasized here is that, similar to all of the other treatments described above, it was necessary to replace the self-stimulatory behavior with another behavior, and not to merely eliminate the behavior by itself.

Specially Assessed Reinforcers

The effect of specially assessed reinforcers on the stereotyped behavior of six students who had autism was analyzed by Dyer (1987). Prior to the treatment sessions, she presented various activities to each student and rated preferred objects based on the following criteria:

1. The student manipulates the object for more than 15 seconds.

2. The student resists when the therapist attempts to take the object away.

3. When the object is placed 1 foot from the student, the student reaches for it within 3 seconds.

4. The student exhibits positive affect while manipulating the object.

5. The student selects the object from a pool of objects meeting the above criteria.

She then compared the use of the above (specially assessed reinforcers) with reinforcers that are typically used with children with autism, and had previously been given to the student and resulted in increases in responding. The typical reinforcers consisted of verbal praise paired with food (i.e., potato chips, candy, or juice).

The results of this study revealed that all of the students showed greater decreases in stereotypy and concurrent increases in correct responding and attempts to respond during the specially assessed reinforcer condition, without any type of external suppression of self-stimulation.

These decreases in self-stimulation suggest that powerful external reinforcers may compete with the internal reinforcers provided by self-stimulatory behaviors. Thus, by directly attacking the problem we have been alluding to throughout this article (i.e., self-stimulatory behavior may provide reinforcers that compete with normal reinforcers), it seems possible to conduct a relatively easy, nonaversive treatment procedure to decrease self-stimulation and increase appropriate behaviors in severely handicapped students.

Antecedent Physical Exercise

In our laboratories we have recently looked into the effects of noncontingent antecedent physical exercise on stereotypic behavior and appropriate responding in seven severely handicapped children with autism. Our first study (Kern, Koegel, Dyer, Blew, & Fenton, 1982) showed that brief (15-minute) antecedent jogging periods resulted in lower levels of stereotypic behavior and also produced increases in appropriate play and academic responding. In addition, supplementary measures taken in a classroom setting showed the same trends; on-task behavior increased significantly as did general interest ratings on school tasks.

In a second study (Kern, Koegel, & Dunlap, 1984), we more closely examined the effects of the specific type of physical exercise on the childrens' stereotypic behaviors. We found that 15 minutes of mild exercise (ball playing) had very little or no effect on the childrens' subsequent behaviors.

However, in contrast, 15 minutes of continuous and vigorous exercise (jogging) was always followed by reductions in autistic stereotypic behaviors.

The results of these studies are consistent with those of other studies showing relationships between physical exercise and stereotypic behavior. For example, Watters and Watters (1980) also showed that, following jogging, self-stimulatory behaviors decreased in children who had autism. Additionally, they obtained measures on control groups who did not jog and did not show reductions during the same activities (watching TV or engaging in classroom activities). Further, Ohlsen (1978) found that blind children reduced bodyrocking following vigorous 40-minute daily workouts on exercise equipment.

Evidence of increased and improved respondings in our own data can also be compared with other studies showing similar improvements in cognitive functioning following physical exercise. For example, certain perceptual motor training programs have resulted in significant improvements in visual-motor function (Schaney, Brekke, Landry, & Burke, 1976). Jogging also has been shown to result in significant improvements in psychological test results of psychiatric hospital patients aged from the teens on into the 50s (Dodson & Mullens, 1969). Also, Powell (1974) and Diesfeldt and Diesfeldt-Groenendijk (1977) found significant improvements in the results of two of three cognitive tests in institutionalized geriatric mental patients following physical activity. Finally, Eickelberg, Less, & Engels (1976) found significant increases in learning in passively exercised children who had muscular dystrophy. As a whole, these studies suggest that increases in vigorous physical activity reduce stereotypic and other inappropriate (e.g., off-task) behaviors and simultaneously increase appropriate behaviors.

In addition, the use of such antecedent physical activities has important implications for the ease of management of inappropriate behaviors. That is, long periods of vigilance to detect the occurrence of the behavior and then consequate it are not necessary. Instead, strategically interspersed physical activity classes during the day may promote learning and reduce self-stimulation without further teacher intervention. This is particularly practical in classroom settings that have large groups of children, thereby limiting teaching time and decreasing the likelihood of consistent, immediate, and contingent consequences for inappropriate behaviors.

It is also interesting to consider physiological implications in relation to this research. Many have hypothesized a physiological etiology of autism. Also, we know that physical exercise has a direct effect on changes relating to cardiovascular variables, blood chemistry, oxygen intake, metabolic responses, and so forth. Physiological variables correlating with the behavioral changes we have seen might be a particularly important area for future research (Sahley & Panksepp, 1987). That is, physical exercise classes incorporated into the school curriculum may provide a simple alternative to drug manipulations of blood chemistry and may naturally eliminate or reduce physiological needs for inappropriate self-stimulation.

Sensory Assessment and Extinction

The theory behind sensory extinction involves the notion that if self-stimulation is motivated by its sensory consequences, such as the proprioceptive, auditory, or visual stimulation it produces, then removal of those consequences should cause extinction of the self-stimulation. Procedurally, the process involves identifying the sensory consequence that is maintaining a behavior and then making it so that it no longer provides the reinforcer. For example, Rincover (1978) observed children who engaged in high rates of self-stimulatory behavior. One child would incessantly spin objects, particularly a plate, while cocking his head toward it, apparently listening to it spin. In order to mask the sensory reinforcers, a carpet was placed on top of the child's desk so that spinning the object would not result in auditory stimulation. The results showed that the carpeting almost completely eliminated the child's self-stimulatory behavior.

In a later study, Rincover, Cook, Peoples, and Packard (1979) first applied sensory extinction procedures in order to eliminate the self-stimulation. Then they identified toys that provided the same types of sensory stimulation that the self-stimulation had previously provided and trained the children to play appropriately with the toys. Their data showed an inverse relationship between the self-stimulation and appropriate play that seemed to be relatively durable over a period of several months with no external reinforcers for play or restraints on self-stimulation.

Thus, sensory extinction seems to offer many promises as an excellent nonaversive treatment for self-stimulation. However, there may be significant limitations in many cases. That is, while this procedure may result in complete elimination of self-stimulation in children with only a few well-defined self-stimulatory behaviors, other children do not respond as well. This may be related to the fact that some types of self-stimulation may involve multiple sensory determinants and thus may have to be eliminated by a more elaborate sensory extinction procedure (Rincover et al., 1979). Furthermore, some types of more subtle self-stimulatory behaviors, such as manipulation of the tongue inside of the mouth, might be more difficult to observe and/or mask. Perhaps in these cases one may have to rely more heavily on teaching an alternative appropriate means of obtaining the postulated sensory reinforcer. In any case, with this relatively recent procedure, many children have shown dramatic and durable reductions in their self-stimulation (Devany & Rincover, 1982). Additionally, it may be important to note that the procedure requires very little staff training and thus is both time and cost efficient. This would make it an excellent research area for settings such as classrooms, where a one-to-one ratio is not provided (Devany & Rincover, 1982).

SUMMARY AND LIKELY
AVENUES FOR
FUTURE RESEARCH

It has taken many years of research to successfully teach children who have autism and other severe handicaps. At this point in time, many variables relating to successful and unsuccessful classroom integration have been delineated (Koegel, 1982). As a result, many of the young children who were previously institutionalized are now able to live and interact successfully in a variety of community settings (Dunlap, Koegel, & Koegel, 1984). In earlier years, most research work primarily involved punishment procedures, many of which were quite aversive and painful, to deal with problematic behaviors such as aggression, self-injurious behavior, and self-stimulation.

However, as research is rapidly progressing, many nonaversive treatment avenues that are easily applicable in the community are emerging, often based on the variables identified in the earlier research. These new techniques are based predominantly on the earlier finding that suppression of certain types of self-stimulation (Dunlap et al., 1983) also produces increases in other appropriate means of obtaining sensory input (such as play, speech, social behavior, etc.). Therefore, at this point, the manipulation of numerous antecedent variables seems to be a promising avenue for the treatment of problematic behaviors such as self-stimulation. In addition to providing physical activity classes (Kern et al., 1982; 1984), teaching communicative equivalent phrases (Durand & Carr, 1987), and utilizing sensory extinction procedures (Rincover et al., 1979), researchers are also studying variables related to task manipulation to increase the motivation to learn (Dunlap, 1984; Koegel & Koegel, 1986) and the use of self-monitoring procedures to decrease self-stimulation and self-injurious behavior (see initial studies by Koegel & Koegel, 1986; 1987).

In an overview of all of the research, the most consistent findings relating to the successful remediation of self-stimulation have been that certain types of self-stimulation covary inversely with certain appropriate behaviors, and that the simultaneous manipulation of these appropriate behaviors, often coupled with initial mild response suppression or direct interruption of the self-stimulation seems to provide the most effective treatment strategy. This is true because (a) it is easy to perform such treatments in an educational setting; (b) the treatment directly improves appropriate performance; (c) the treatment may relate to physiological bases of the behavior and/or the reinforcement of the behavior; and (d) the treatment offers the most generalized durable results in community settings shown to date. Thus, although the treatment of self-stimulation still does not seem to be completely developed at this point in time, the identification of variables related to it now offers a level of optimism and current treatment application that was not feasible before, and the future seems likely to continue to produce significant improvements.

REFERENCES

Barkley, R. A., & Zupnick, S. (1976). Reduction of stereotypic body contortions using physical restraint and DRO. *Journal of Behavior Therapy and Experimental Psychiatry, 7,* 167–170.

Barrett, R. P., & Shapiro, E. S. (1980). Treatment of stereotyped hair-pulling with overcorrection: A case study with long term follow-up. *Journal of Behavioral and Experimental Psychiatry, 11,* 317–320.

Baumeister, A. A., & Forehand, R. (1972). Effects of contingent shock and verbal command on bodyrocking of retardates. *Journal of Clinical Psychology, 28,* 586–590.

Berkson G. (1965). Stereotyped movements of mental defectives. VI. No effect of amphetamine or a barbituate. *Perceptual and Motor Skills, 21,* 698.

Coleman, R. S., Whitman, T. L., & Johnson, M. R. (1979). Suppression of self-stimulatory behavior of a profoundly retarded boy across staff and settings: An assessment of situational generalization. *Behavior Therapy, 10,* 266–280.

Devany, J., & Rincover, A. (1982). Self-stimulatory behavior and sensory reinforcement. In R. L. Koegel, A. Rincover, & A. L. Egel (Eds.), *Educating and understanding autistic children.* San Diego: College-Hill Press.

Diesfeldt, H. F. A., Diesfeldt-Groenendijk, H. (1977). Improving cognitive performance in psychogeriatric patients. *Age and Aging, 6,* 58–64.

Dodson, L. C., & Mullens, W. R. (1969). Some effects of jogging on psychiatric hospital patients. *American Correctional Therapy Journal, 5,* 130–134.

Doke, L. A., & Epstein, L. H. (1975). Oral overcorrection: Side effects and extended applications. *Journal of Experimental Child Psychology, 20,* 496–511.

Dunlap, G. (1984). The influence of task variation and maintenance tasks on the learning and affect of autistic children. *Journal of Experimental Child Psychology, 37,* 41–64.

Dunlap, G., Dyer, K., & Koegel, R. L. (1983). Autistic self-stimulation. *American Journal of Mental Deficiency, 88,* 194–202.

Dunlap, G., Koegel, R. L., Johnson, J., & O'Neill, R. E. (1987). Maintaining performance of autistic clients in community settings with delayed contingencies. *Journal of Applied Behavior Analysis, 20,* 185–191.

Dunlap, G., Koegel, R. L., Koegel, L. K. (1984). Continuity of treatment: Toilet training in multiple community settings. *Journal of the Association for Persons with Severe Handicaps, 9,* 134–141.

Durand, V. M., & Carr, E. G. (1987). Social influences on "self-stimulatory" behavior: Analysis and treatment application. *Journal of Applied Behavior Analysis, 20,* 119–132.

Dyer, K. (1987). The competition of autistic stereotyped behavior with usual and specially assessed reinforcers. *Research in Developmental Disabilities, 8,* 607–626.

Eickelberg, W. W. B., Less, M., & Engels, W. C. (1976). Respiratory, cardiac and learning changes in exercised muscular dystrophic children. *Perceptual and Motor Skills, 43,* 66.

Epstein, L. H., Doke, L. A., Sajwaj, T. E., Sorrell, S., & Rimmer, B. (1974). Generality and side effects of overcorrection. *Journal of Applied Behavior Analysis, 7,* 385–390.

Favell, J. E. (1973). Reduction of stereotypies by reinforcement of toy play. *Mental Retardation, 11,* 21–23.

Foxx, R. M., & Azrin, N. H. (1973). The elimination of autistic self-stimulatory behavior by overcorrection. *Journal of Applied Behavior Analysis, 6,* 1–14.

Foxx, R. M., & Bechtel, D. R. (1982). Overcorrection. *Progress in Behavior Modification, 13,* 227–288.

Freeman, B. J., Moss, D., Somerset, T., & Ritvo, E. R. (1977). Thumbsucking in an autistic child overcome by overcorrection. *Journal of Behavior Therapy and Experimental Psychiatry, 8,* 211–212.

Greene, R. J., Hoats, D. L., & Hornick, A. J. (1970). Music distortion: A new technique for behavior modification. *The Psychological Record, 20,* 107–109.

Harris, S. L., & Wolchik, S. A. (1979). Suppression of self-stimulation: Three alternative strategies. *Journal of Applied Behavior Analysis, 12,* 185–198.

Hobbs, S., & Goswick, R. (1977). Behavioral treatment of self-stimulation: An experimentation of alternatives to physical punishment. *Journal of Clinical Child Psychology, 6,* 20–23.

Kern, L., Koegel, R. L., & Dunlap, G. (1984). The influence of vigorous versus mild exercise on autistic stereotyped behaviors. *Journal of Autism and Developmental Disorders, 14,* 57–67.

Kern, L., Koegel, R. L., Dyer, K., Blew, P. A., & Fenton, L. R. (1982). The effects of physical exercise on self-stimulation and appropriate responding in autistic children. *Journal of Autism and Developmental Disorders, 12,* 399–419.

Koegel, R. L. (1982). *How to integrate autistic and other severely handicapped children into a classroom.* Lawrence, KS: H & H Enterprises, Inc.

Koegel, R. L., & Covert, A. (1972). The relationship of self-stimulation to learning in autistic children. *Journal of Applied Behavior Analysis, 5,* 381–387.

Koegel, R. L., Firestone, P. B., Kramme, K. W., & Dunlap, G. (1974). Increasing spontaneous play by suppressing self-stimulation in autistic children. *Journal of Applied Behavior Analysis, 7,* 521–528.

Koegel, R. L., & Koegel, L. K. (1986). Promoting generalized treatment gains through direct instruction of self-monitoring skills. *Direct Instruction News, 5,* 13–15.

Koegel, R. L., & Koegel, L. K. (1987). Generalization issues in the treatment of autism. *Seminars in Speech and Language, 8,* 241–256.

Koegel, R. L., O'Dell, M., & Dunlap, G. (in press). Producing speech use in nonverbal autistic children by reinforcing attempts. *Journal of Autism and Developmental Disorders.*

Koegel, R. L., O'Dell, M. C., & Koegel, L. K. (1987). A natural language teaching paradigm for nonverbal autistic children. *Journal of Autism and Developmental Disorders, 17,* 187–200.

LaGrow, S. J., & Repp, A. C. (1984). Stereotypic responding: A review of intervention research. *American Journal of Mental Deficiency, 88,* 595–609.

LaVigna, G. W., & Donnellan, A. M. (1986). *Alternatives to punishment: Solving behavior problems with non-aversive strategies.* New York: Irvington Publishers, Inc.

Lovaas, O. I., Freitag, G., Kinder, M. I., Rubenstein, B. D., Schaeffer, B., & Simmons, J. Q. (1966). Establishment of social reinforcers in schizophrenic children using food. *Journal of Experimental Child Psychology, 4,* 109–125.

Lovaas, O. I., Litrownik, A., & Mann, R. (1971). Response latencies to auditory stimuli in autistic children engaged in self-stimulatory behavior. *Behaviour Research and Therapy, 9,* 39–49.

Lovaas, O. I., Newsom, C., & Hickman, C. (1987). Self-stimulatory behavior and perceptual reinforcement. *Journal of Applied Behavior Analysis, 20,* 45–68.

Lovaas, O. I., Varni, J. W., Koegel, R. L., & Lorsch, N. (1977). Some observations on the nonextinguishability of children's speech. *Child Development, 48,* 1121–1127.

Luiselli, J. K., Helfen, C. S., Pemberton, B. W., & Reisman, J. (1977). The elimination of a child's in-class masturbation by overcorrection and reinforcement. *Journal of Behavior Therapy and Experimental Psychiatry, 8,* 201–204.

Luiselli, J. K., Pemberton, B. W., & Helfen, C. S. (1978). Effects and side effects of a brief overcorrection procedure in reducing multiple self-stimulatory behaviour: A single case analysis. *Journal of Mental Deficiency Research, 22,* 287–293.

Marholin II, D., Touchette, P. E., & Stewart, R. M. (1979). Withdrawal of chronic chlorpromazine medication: An experimental analysis. *Journal of Applied Behavior Analysis, 12,* 159–171.

Martin, J., Weller, S., & Matson, J. (1977). Eliminating object-transferring by a profoundly retarded female by overcorrection. *Psychological Reports, 40,* 779–782.

150   SEVERE PROBLEMS

Matson, J. L., & Stephens, R. M. (1981). Overcorrection treatment of stereotyped behaviors. *Behavior Modification, 5,* 491–502.

Neef, N. A., Iwata, B. A., & Page, T. J. (1980). The effects of interspersal training versus high density reinforcement on spelling acquisition and performance. *Journal of Applied Behavior Analysis, 13,* 153–158.

Newsom, C. D., Carr, E., & Lovaas, O. I (1977). Experimental analysis and modification of autistic behavior. In R. S. Davidson (Ed.), *Experimental analysis of clinical phenomena.* New York: Gardner Press.

Ohlsen, R. L. (1978). Control of bodyrocking in the blind through use of vigorous exercise. *Journal of Instructional Psychology, 5,* 19–22.

Ollendick, T. H., Shapiro, E. S., & Barrett, R. P. (1981). Reducing stereotypic behaviors: An analysis of treatment procedures utilizing an alternating treatments design. *Behavior Therapy, 12,* 570–577.

Pendergrass, V. E. (1972). Timeout from positive reinforcement following persistent, high-rate behavior in retardates. *Journal of Applied Behavior Analysis, 5,* 85–91.

Powell, R. R. (1974). Psychological effects of exercise therapy upon institutionalized geriatric mental patients. *Journal of Gerontology, 29,* 157–161.

Repp, A. C., & Barton, L. E. (1980). Naturalistic observations of institutionalized retarded persons: A comparison of licensure decisions and behavioral observations. *Journal of Applied Behavior Analysis, 13,* 333–341.

Repp, A. C., Dietz, S. M., & Dietz, D. E. (1976). Reducing inappropriate behaviors in classrooms and in individual sessions through DRO schedules of reinforcement. *Mental Retardation, 14,* 11–15.

Rincover, A. (1978). Sensory extinction: A procedure for eliminating self-stimulatory behavior in developmentally disabled children. *Journal of Abnormal Child Psychology, 6,* 299–310.

Rincover, A., Cook, R., Peoples, A., & Packard, D. (1979). Sensory extinction and sensory reinforcement principles for programming multiple adaptive behavior change. *Journal of Applied Behavior Analysis, 12,* 221–233.

Rincover, A., Newsom, C. D., Lovaas, O. I., & Koegel, R. L. (1977). Some motivational properties of sensory reinforcement in psychotic children. *Journal of Experimental Child Psychology, 24,* 312–323.

Risley, T. (1968). The effects and side effects of punishing the autistic behaviors of a deviant child. *Journal of Applied Behavior Analysis, 1,* 21–34.

Roberts, P., Iwata, B. A., McSween, T. E., & Desmond, Jr., E. F. (1979). An analysis of overcorrection movements. *American Journal of Mental Deficiency, 83,* 588–594.

Rutter M. (1966). Prognosis. In J. K. Wing (Ed.), *Early childhood autism.* Oxford: Pergamon Press.

Sachs, D. A. (1973). The efficacy of time-out procedures in a variety of behavior problems. *Journal of Behavior Therapy and Experimental Psychiatry, 4,* 237–242.

Sahley, T. L., & Panksepp, J. (1987). Brain opioids and autism: An updated analysis of possible linkages. *Journal of Autism and Developmental Disorders, 17,* 201–216.

Schaney, Z., Brekke, B., Landry, R., & Burke, J. (1976). Effects of a perceptual-motor training program on kindergarten children. *Perceptual and Motor Skills, 43,* 428–430.

Schopler, E. (1986). Treatment abuse and its reduction. *Journal of Autism and Developmental Disorders, 16,* 99–104.

Shapiro, E. S., Barrett, R. P., & Ollendick, T. H. (1980). A comparison of physical restraint and positive practice overcorrection in treating stereotypic behavior. *Behavior Therapy, 11,* 227–233.

Solnick, J. V., Rincover, A., & Peterson, C. R. (1977). Some determinants of the reinforcing and punishing effects of timeout. *Journal of Applied Behavior Analysis, 10,* 415–424.

Watters, R. G., & Watters, W. E. (1980). Decreasing self-stimulatory behavior with physical exercise in a group of autistic boys. *Journal of Autism and Developmental Disorders, 10,* 379–387.

Winterling, V., Dunlap, G., & O'Neill, R. E. (1987). The influence of task variation on the aberrant behaviors of autistic students. *Education and Treatment of Children, 10,* 105–119.

Yarbrough, E., Sentat, U., Perel, I., Webster, C., & Lombardi, R. (1987). Effects of fenfluramine on autistic individuals residing in a state developmental center. *Journal of Autism and Developmental Disorders, 17,* 303–314.

Training
Concerns

Behavioral Parent Training

Andrew L. Egel
and
Michael D. Powers
University of Maryland, College Park

A View of the Past and Suggestions for the Future

Providing parents with the skills to affect their children's behavior has been a feature of applied behavior analysis for over two decades. During this time, parents of both handicapped and nonhandicapped children have been taught (using several different methodologies) a variety of skills to change an array of behaviors. The inclusion of parents as intervention agents was logical because they had the opportunities to teach their children in many more and diverse settings than were available to teachers or clinicians. Numerous investigations with parents of both handicapped and nonhandicapped children have supported this belief by demonstrating that parents can be very effective in changing/maintaining their child's behavior (Bernal, Klinnert, & Schultz, 1980; Dangel & Polster, 1984; Forehand & King, 1977; Hall, Christler, Cranston, & Tucker, 1970; Harris, Wolchik, & Milch, 1983; O'Dell, Krug, Patterson, & Faustman, 1980; Patterson & Reid, 1973; Schreibman, Koegel, Mills, & Burke, 1984).

The importance of including parents as intervention agents was demonstrated very clearly by Lovaas and his colleagues in their longitudinal study of 20 autistic children (Lovaas, Koegel, Simmons, & Long, 1973). Four years after the original treatment program was discontinued, the authors found that the only children who continued to improve were those whose parents had received training in behavioral principles. In stark contrast, treatment gains were not maintained in children institutionalized following training or who remained with parents who had not received training.

This chapter provides an overview of past and present research on parent training. In the first section, we review the methods used to teach parents, the skills taught most frequently, and the outcomes of such train-

Acknowledgments.   Preparation of this chapter was supported in part by a grant from the U.S. Office of Education, No. G008630278. Both authors contributed equally to this chapter. Order of authorship was determined alphabetically.

ing. In the second section, we discuss shortcomings of traditional models of parent training, changes that may be necessary to address them, and questions that still remain.

A variety of programs/models have been developed for training parents and are reviewed by Polster and Dangel (1984). In general, parents have been taught behavioral principles and procedures such as reinforcement, punishment, error correction, prompting, shaping, chaining, and/or appropriate instructional delivery. Training methods have included (either separately or, more typically, in combination): discussion and written materials (Arnold, Sturgis, & Forehand, 1977; Fowler, Johnson, Whitman, & Zukotynski, 1978; Friman, Barnard, Altman, & Wolf, 1986; Kelly, Embry, & Baer, 1979); behavioral rehearsal and feedback (Forehand & King, 1977; Friman et al., 1986; Peed, Roberts, & Forehand, 1977); and modeling procedures both *in vivo* and through videotapes (Koegel, Glahn, & Nieminen, 1978; O'Dell, Krug, O'Quin, & Kasnetz, 1980; O'Dell, Mahoney, Horton, & Turner, 1979). Whether or not any individual method or a specific combination of these procedures is more effective and/or efficient in training parents has been addressed in several investigations (Eyberg & Matarazzo, 1980; Heifetz, 1977; Koegel et al., 1978; O'Dell et al., 1979; O'Dell, O'Quin, Alford, O'Briant, Bradlyn, & Giebenhain, 1982). Although the results of many of the studies should be interpreted cautiously because of potential methodological shortcomings (e.g., use of parent observation data, variation in presentation format and/or time; O'Dell, 1985), the data suggest that, typically, modeling (either *in vivo* or through videotapes) is more effective than written manuals or verbal discussion in teaching behavioral principles to parents. Despite this general trend, O'Dell et al. (1982) found no significant differences between written, videotaped, or *in vivo* training methods when they taught parents how to reinforce appropriately. The results from this study and others suggest that the effectiveness or ineffectiveness of specific training procedures may be a function of variables other than the procedure per se. For example, the relationship between parents' education level and the reading level of written material may influence the usefulness of a manual or other written material. Similarly, the effectiveness of modeling (*in vivo* or videotaped) as a training strategy can be influenced by variety of variables including status, age, and sex of the model.

Training procedures have typically been presented in one of three formats: individual, group, or a combination of individual and group. Whether one format is more effective than another has been evaluated in several investigations (Christensen, Johnson, Phillips, & Glasgow, 1980; Kovitz, 1976). Although these studies used different sized groups and did not necessarily conduct them in the same fashion, objective measures of changes in parent behavior demonstrated that group and individual instruction were equally effective. Additional data on the relationship between training format and factors such as the amount of training time involved with each approach, severity of the child's behavioral excesses and deficits, and parent/therapist satisfaction with the type of training are necessary before trainers will be able to select a format based on child and family characteristics. However, the data on training parents in groups are promising and, to a large extent, consistent with the literature on group versus individual instruction in the classroom (Favell & Reid, 1984).

Regardless of the format or procedures used, most programs focus on teaching parents a general set of skills (based on behavioral principles) that enable them to respond to a variety of child behaviors (Polster & Dangle, 1984). As part of a multicomponent study, Koegel et al. (1978) compared this approach with one that taught parents how to teach one specific behavior at a time. Their results demonstrated that teaching parents to modify individual behaviors was an effective approach for changing that specific behavior; however, parents' teaching abilities generalized to novel tasks only after they received training in general behavior management procedures.

Overall, there is clear evidence that the majority of parents can be successfully taught a variety of skills, and that they can use these abilities to teach their children functional skills as well as to reduce behavioral excesses. Parent training thus represents one of the major achievements of the behavioral approach to working with families.

Despite the accomplishments of parent training models, several findings were disconcerting. Two of the more serious, interrelated concerns were: generalization and maintenance of skills; and why some families were not benefiting from the training. Several authors have evaluated the maintenance of parent training gains with parents whose children exhibit a wide variety of behavioral deficiencies and/or excesses (Baker, Heifetz, & Murphy, 1980; Baum & Forehand, 1981; Forehand, Rogers, McMahon, Wells, & Griest, 1981; Forehand, Sturgis, et al., 1979; Griest, Forehand, & Wells, 1981; Harris, 1986; Harris, Wolchik, & Weitz, 1981; Holmes, Hemsley, Rickett, & Likierman, 1982; Wahler, 1980). Overall, the results are not consistent: some studies demonstrated maintenance of child and parent behavior; others have shown maintenance of child or parent behavior; and in some, treatment gains have not been maintained. Furthermore, the reliance on parent report/interview data, different models of training, and different subject populations makes it difficult to evaluate the extent to which parents and children maintain what they have been taught.

The above findings, and concerns about families for whom parent training programs were not successful, have resulted in efforts to identify variables associated with the findings. Research has demonstrated that variables such as socioeconomic level (McMahon, Forehand, Griest, & Wells, 1981; Wahler & Afton, 1980; Webster-Stratton, 1985); marital conflict (Bernal et al., 1980); single parenthood (Strain, Young, & Horowitz, 1981); parental depression (McMahon et al., 1981; Griest et al., 1981); and insularity (Wahler, 1980; Wahler & Dumas, 1984) have all been related to negative parent training outcomes.

Snell and Beckman-Brindley (1984) noted that the effects of these variables may be exacerbated in families with children who are severely handicapped. These families are vulnerable to a high level of psychological stress that may not only detract from their ability to meet the child's needs, but also may result in maladaptive functioning of the family as a whole. Sources of stress include the initial reaction to diagnosis, uncertainty about the child's future, extensive caretaking responsibilities, financial burdens, social isolation, and difficulties negotiating the maze of medical, social, and educational agencies involved with the child. As a result, it may be more difficult for parents of severely handicapped children to continue using the strategies taught during parent training once formal sessions have been completed (Harris et al., 1981; Holmes et al., 1982).

As previously noted, most parent training programs focused on providing parents with a generalized set of skills to teach and/or remediate discrete behaviors. Evaluation typically involved measuring changes in parent and/ or child behavior. How the family functioned as an interactive system was, in most cases, treated as a side issue unrelated to the training process. Thus, a body of information on family functioning was unavailable to evaluate why parents did not acquire or maintain the use of the teaching strategies, or why children did not improve (either at all or at the same rate) over time. This has led to the recent acknowledgement by numerous researchers that parent training as traditionally implemented is insufficient for some families if lasting change is to occur (Dadds, Sanders, & James, 1987; Griest & Forehand, 1982; Harris, 1982, 1988; Kaiser & Fox, 1986; Koegel, Schreibman, Johnson, O'Neill, & Dunlap, 1984; Lutzker, McGimsey, McRae, & Campbell, 1983; Powers & Bruey, 1988; Rios & Gutierrez, 1986; Turnbull, Brotherson, & Summers, 1986; Winton, 1986). These investigators have just begun to address the need for expanding services so that behavioral parent training assesses, implements, and evaluates problems related to the family structure, family relationships, and the lifecycle.

CONCEPTUALIZATION OF THE
FAMILY AS A SYSTEM

Observations of behavioral psychologists (Harris, 1983; Patterson & Fleishman, 1979; Powers & Bruey, 1988) and special educators (Turnbull et al., 1986; Winton, 1986) about the needs of families who have severely handicapped members converge on several important points: (a) families have multiple needs extending well beyond the education of their child(ren); (b) these needs vary according to the age of the child(ren) and the position of the family within the life cycle; (c) assessment of these needs and measurement of outcomes may require different models than those in common use; and (d) too many intervention efforts are characterized by a *unidimensional* approach to helping the child, approaches that fail to understand the child with a severe handicap within his or her relevant social, cultural, familial, and historical contexts. The equivocal results of apparently sound intervention plans with families of children with severe handicaps (Snell & Beckman-Brindley, 1984) argue for closer scrutiny of systemic factors promoting or impeding change. The challenge becomes one of identifying a conceptual framework for understanding the process of change in the family of the person with a severe handicap, and of applying that understanding to the needs of families at a given point in time and across the lifecycle.

We believe that systems models (Miller, 1978; von Bertalanffy, 1968) for explaining human behavior offer a theoretical framework compatible with the needs of the person who is assessing, treating, and evaluating outcomes of families of children with severe handicaps (Powers, 1988). More importantly, a systems approach to behavioral parent training expands the utility of this intervention method in important ways by acknowledging relevant aspects of a family's ecology, helping to predict potential sources of resistance, identifying family risk factors, and by guiding intervention.

RELEVANT CONCEPTS

A systems approach to behavioral parent training incorporates the behavior analytic model into a broader intervention approach that addresses the structure and functioning of the entire family system. Although the value inherent in considering the family's ecology may be apparent, we must stress that for the present such a model has heuristic value only. We are aware of only a very few empirical investigations of the effect of behavioral parent training on the family system or on such factors as family cohesion, adaptability, or perceived self-efficacy (Schreibman et al., 1984). Thus, despite its intuitive appeal, much work remains to be done to provide the empirical basis for the integration of behavioral and systems models in parent training.

Although a discussion of the fundamental concepts of systems theory is beyond the scope of this paper, we would like to highlight certain features of a systems approach that we have found useful.

Self-perpetuation

A system, be it a couple, family, or sibling group, has self-perpetuating properties. People within a system learn to engage in behaviors that are most likely to result in reinforcement (either positive or negative). These behaviors may be maladaptive yet firmly established in a person's repertoire by their history of reinforcement. Consider, for example, a situation in which tantrum behavior is maintained by parent attention. The attention results in temporary cessation of the tantrum (thus negatively reinforcing the parent's response); however, it subsequently reoccurs at a higher rate and/or intensity. These types of behavior patterns are typically self-perpetuating because they are "successful" (i.e., reinforced) and as a result can affect other subsystems in the family when the same or similar responses are used in other situations. Parent training outcomes can be affected unless the trainer and parents select a target behavior that is likely to respond very quickly to an intervention that does not immediately require extensive changes in the family interactional patterns.

Boundaries

A second contribution of systems theory is the delineation of subsystems and the identification of boundaries between these subsystems. When examining the family unit, four basic subsystems can be described: the spousal subsystem, the parental subsystem, the sibling subsystem, and the intergenerational or extended family subsystem. Ideally, the boundaries between these subsystems should be well defined, where all family members have clearly acknowledged roles as per their inclusion in a given subsystem. Often, however, boundaries become diffused: roles are unclear and interactions reflect enmeshment and/or disengagement.

The child with a severe handicap has the potential to threaten boundaries insofar as he or she does not fit neatly into the sibling subsystem (Harris, 1983). For example, the child's healthy siblings may view themselves as half siblings, half parent. They attempt to include the sibling with a severe handicap while providing whatever extra supervision is required, potentially taking on a role that Minuchin (1974) terms the "parental child," a role that may be detrimental to their own psychological development.

Boundaries between parents and offspring are often affected by the presence of a child with a severe handicap (Featherstone, 1980; Harris & Powers, 1984). The child's need for heightened supervision and attention may lead some parents to become overinvolved, thus creating an enmeshed relationship. Conversely, the child's aggressive or self-injurious behavior may prompt his or her parents to become excessively disengaged. Meanwhile, the nondisabled offspring are caught in this imbalance of relationships.

Finally, boundaries between the family and the rest of the world are frequently too rigid when a child with a severe handicap is present. Community activities may be infrequent because of the child's inappropriate behaviors, or family members may feel "too different" to be part of their friends' community (Featherstone, 1980; Holroyd & McArthur, 1976) and may begin identifying themselves solely as "a family with a handicapped member."

Transitions

A third application of systems theory is that the family is in perpetual transition. For example, the transactional patterns, needs, and community involvement of a family with two toddlers are markedly different than those seen in the same family 10 years later, after the toddlers have reached adolescence. Each transition in the family life cycle inevitably produces stress on the family system because of the changes that transitions require. Moreover, the very process of receiving information, evaluating it, and deciding on its applicability to the system's well being involve periodic transitional crises that promote growth. Of course, transitions for families with a severely handicapped child are likely to be more stressful. For example, the transition to adolescence may in new problems (i.e., stress) for most families; however, it is particularly difficult for families in which the adolescent cannot/does not understand the internal changes that are occurring.

THE FAMILY
LIFE CYCLE

The assumption that systems are self-perpetuating and evolutionary implies a developmental progression over time of family functioning. In considering families with a member who is severely handicapped, it is helpful to consider their position on this developmental continuum as a means of understanding those life events that may create situational, transitional stress.

Having a child with a severe handicap affects the evolution of the family life cycle. For example, the mother of a 16-year-old daughter with severe mental retardation has parental obligations that no longer concern her peer group (e.g., finding a babysitter). Similarly, the child with a severe handicap rarely achieves the degree of independence necessary to live on his/her own. Consequently, when their peers are planning weddings or anticipating grandchildren, the parents of a young adult with a severe handicap may be exploring the possibility of residential placement.

Four major stages of the life cycle of families with a developmentally disabled member can be delineated: preschool, school age, adolescence, and adulthood (Harris & Powers, 1984). Transitional events that are either different from the norm (e.g., the birth of a child with a handicap) or temporally delayed (e.g., the child first learning to walk at 27 months) are disruptive to family functioning. Numerous events that produce stress across the life cycle have been identified, including obtaining a diagnosis; first telling extended family members of the child's disability; entering the child in school; finding and interacting with medical specialists; missed transitional events having religious or ethnic significance (e.g., Bar Mitzvah); the emergence of sexuality during adolescence; and issues related to the lack of independence into adulthood (Harris & Powers, 1984; Mesibov, 1983; Turnbull & Winton, 1984).

CHARACTERISTICS OF A SYSTEMS APPROACH TO BEHAVIORAL PARENT TRAINING

Three characteristics of a systems approach can be described: ecological sensitivity, attention to family process, and awareness of interrelatedness of different levels of the family system and component subsystems.

Ecological Sensitivity

For a parent trainer to teach a family to implement a behavioral treatment program successfully and maintain it over time, there must be explicit recognition that proposed change in one part of the family system will affect other parts of the family system, as well as systems beyond the family (e.g., school).

Predicting these covariations is very difficult. However, this process may be facilitated if the parent trainer assesses prior to intervention the extent to which the proposed program fits the structure of the family. Variables to assess include, but are not limited to family management style; rules for participation; responsibilities of members of the family; cultural, ethnic, or religious values; socioeconomic status; and financial, physical, and material resources available. Powers and Handleman (1984) provided a more extensive discussion of these factors.

To maintain sensitivity to ecological issues and thereby facilitate maintenance of systemic change Barber, Barber, and Clark (1983) recommended
consideration of the following:

1. Careful determination of family needs in the community. Respon-
   siveness to these needs and an awareness of the interrelationship
   of basic needs to larger service delivery needs is important.

2. Determination of the acceptability of services currently available.

3. Development of an understanding of how the family would like
   things to be by having them identify what in the environment must
   change (i.e., target behaviors) for this desirable state to exist.

4. Identification of available and potential interventions along the continuum of *less restrictive* to *more restrictive* to address discrepancies
   between the current and desirable circumstances, considering the
   reasonableness of cost, both financial and in time spent, of these
   options.

5. Where possible, incorporate community members and relevant organizations (e.g., schools) into the treatment planning process in
   order to develop broad based support and to access existing community resources.

6. Plan in detail for training, implementation, generalization, and
   evaluation of the intervention by all involved.

When establishing a new intervention program or substantially expanding an old one, professionals must recognize that the program is not being
introduced into a vacuum. Rather, the family has been responding (with
varying degrees of success of failure) with the help of existing service
delivery options (Rosenberg, Reppucci, & Linney, 1983) or their own informal service networks (Kleinman, Eisenberg, & Good, 1978). As such, new
treatment programs enter an existing ecology and their implementation
may be disrupted by the contingencies established through previous (formal
and informal) treatment programs.

It is erroneous to assume that simply because a treatment program is
developed by learned persons, it will be both appropriate and accepted by
the family. Initial acceptance and long term maintenance of new interventions may be jeopardized if professionals proposing new treatment programs do not recognize that the response requirements of a new intervention may be inconsistent with the history of reinforcement that exists within
the family system, and incorporate salient aspects of social and political
ecologies (e.g., existing family structure; presence of very young siblings,
working/nonworking mothers and fathers, work hours, child care responsibilities, etc.) into their intervention plans.

Attention to Family Process

The evolution of families is heavily influenced by ideological, social, moral, political, and economic issues. Unfortunately, parent trainers often fail to recognize the importance of these elements in the planning, implementation, and evaluation phases of program development. Particularly important aspects of family process to consider include who makes decisions, where the alliances are between family members, the stability or dysfunction of various key subsystems (spousal, marital, sibling), the role of cultural and ethnic factors on family process, and the effect of extended family and social networks on family process. Not only must professionals be competent at applying behavior analytic procedures to increase desirable behavior and reduce problematic behavior, but they must also be skilled observers of family process and the effect of family process on the target behavior(s) of concern.

Awareness of Interrelationships

Attention to the interaction between a family and the environment is critical for program success (Bronfenbrenner, 1986; Mash, 1987). Unfortunately, researchers have only recently included the measurement of person-environment interaction and intraindividual variables in their work (Evans, 1985; Moos, 1979).

Interrelationships can be identified at several levels: behavioral, ecological, and historical. At the behavioral level, the relationship between targeted and nontargeted (collateral) behaviors must be considered because unplanned positive and negative effects of treatment are sometimes observed with individuals with severe handicaps (Barbrack, 1985; Evans, 1985; Neef, Shafer, Egel, Cataldo, & Parrish, 1983; Nordquist, 1971; Russo, Cataldo, & Cushing, 1981). These response covariations or interrelationships occur because several behaviors may exist as part of a single response class, whereby changes in the antecedent or consequent stimuli for one behavior will trigger a change in other behaviors.

The ecological level is concerned with the environmental constraints within which a current or proposed intervention exists, with special emphasis on the "goodness-of-fit" between the philosophies and values of the family and those of the person proposing the intervention. For example, ecological components for analysis of a child with autism and her family would include the family's readiness for change (Powers & Handleman, 1984), the family's technical skill in managing their child's behavior (Harris, 1984), the presence and capabilities of siblings (Lobato & Barrera, 1988), the family's response to raising an autistic child (Harris, 1982), the present position of the child within the family's life cycle (Harris & Powers, 1984), and the family's cultural and ethnic heritage (Powers, 1986a).

Community factors must also be considered when examining ecological interrelationships. Identification of commonalities between the family and the community by the parent trainer facilitates this process. Few human service organizations have the financial, human, technical, and physical resources to meet the extensive needs of their clients. Coordination and resource networking with other agencies increases the comprehensiveness of services available, reduces duplication of efforts, and actively integrates various constituencies from within the community into the service delivery process (Powers, 1986b).

Historical interrelationships represent points of convergence between a family's reinforcement history and its predicted or actual response to a new intervention. By addressing the relevant historical context in social, political, and economic domains (with special emphasis on how these three interrelated domains have impacted upon the family's prior attempts at change), the professional avoids a myopic view of the family's behavior (Reppucci & Saunders, 1983). For example, knowledge that a family's historical response to outside professionals proposing change is to initially engage in avoidance behaviors and/or respond with behaviors that were reinforced previously provides the professional with a realistic understanding of how to proceed in the intervention process.

BROADENING THE GOALS
OF BEHAVIOR
PARENT TRAINING

Given the wealth of empirical evidence supporting the efficacy of behavior analytic procedures in training parents of children with severe handicaps, it is essential to develop specific, behaviorally based treatment programs addressing socially valid problems. Equally important, however, is the need to expand the intervention process to include goals that address family structure and functioning. A systems approach underscores the importance of ecological factors that promote and support family wellness. The following six goals represent additional areas for assessment and intervention for the professional adopting a systems approach to behavioral parent training. Taken together, these goals assist in the development and maintenance of normal family process across the lifespan.

Facilitating a Healthy Response to Diagnosis

Knowledge of potential affective responses to diagnosis will help the professional to label behavior and affective responses of family members and to place such reactions within a normal developmental context.

Facilitating Service Access and Coordination

The professional's role as liaison to medical, social support, educational, legal, and financial services is a crucial one. By facilitating coordination, consistency, and continuity of services, the professional can gradually transfer his or her knowledge of community services to the family.

Facilitating Development of Parent Advocacy Skills

The mobile nature of American society and the periodic nature of developmental transitions across the lifespan argue for the importance of families learning to advocate for the child with a severe handicap. The professional's role in this process is to empower the family. The professional must move from the position of direct advocate, trainer in advocacy methods, liaison with other professionals and agencies, and pathfinder for existing community services to serve as a consultant in the advocacy process. In so doing, the professional will facilitate the development of family advocacy networks.

Facilitating Structural Balance Within the Family System

The needs of a child with a severe handicap can place excessive demands on both individual family members and the various subsystems within the family. While it is not possible to speak of an "ideal family," it would seem important that certain family structures be supported in counseling. These include the maintenance of role boundaries between parental and sibling subsystem, and the maintenance of a healthy relationship within the marital subsystem. Throughout, the professional's goal is to help the family change dysfunctional organizational patterns.

Promoting Functional Forms of Family Organization

Irrespective of its source, added stress can lead to the establishment of dysfunctional forms of behavior in the nuclear and extended family. In treating families of a child with a severe handicap, professionals must be aware of several potential forms of family dysfunction and be prepared to address them. These include:

1. Cross-generational coalitions may form whereby members of different subsystems work against a common good by joining forces to maintain or advance a particular position. For example, a father and his parents may hold fast to the position that a child with autism will not profit from appropriate limit setting and refuse to set limits, thereby isolating the dissenting mother and disrupting parental and marital subsystem functioning. Unless the parent trainer recognizes this pattern and responds to it, s/he would experience considerable difficulty securing family cooperation on a consistent basis.

2. Hierarchical conflicts between the grandparents and their own child may occur. For example, the mother or father of the handicapped child may not have achieved a sufficient level of differentiation from her or his own family of origin to allow for the healthy development of a separate family system.

3. Parental subsystem conflict leading to disagreement and inconsistency in the treatment of the child.

4. Sibling subsystem dysfunction because of role diffusion of other children (e.g., an oldest daughter becoming a "parental child") or exclusion of other children from significant amounts of parental attention because of parent overinvolvement with the child with a severe handicap.

Facilitating the Development and Maintenance of Social Networks

Embarrassment, fear of rejection by family or community, or the rigors of managing a child with a severe handicap may limit the social contacts of a family. In its most dysfunctional form, the family assumes the primary perception of itself as "a family with a handicapped member" and restricts social contact to other families with handicapped members or to activities revolving around the handicapped child's needs. Such perceptions have reverberating effects on all subsystems. The seminal work of Speck and Attneave (1973) on family networks has considerable relevance here. Families of children with severe handicaps need to maintain open and active networks with community providers of the services needed for themselves and their child. In addition, they must participate in those social networks available to community members without handicapped children. As mentioned previously, the professionals conducting parent training should serve a facilitative role in this process.

IMPLICATIONS OF A
SYSTEMS APPROACH FOR
EVALUATING BEHAVIORAL
PARENT TRAINING

The problem of assessment in psychology and education is one of identifying the appropriate methodology for observing the unit of analysis one is interested in. For those conducting more traditional behavioral parent training, two units of analysis are prominent: child behavior and parent behavior directly related to intervening on the child behavior(s) of interest. Both of these require individual levels of analysis. Expanding parent training to a systems approach requires assessment and intervention efforts at additional levels of the family system: dyadic (e.g., parent-child, husband-wife); and group (e.g., family ecology, community resources). However, as Mash (1984; 1987) noted, the ability to *conceptualize* the child and the family as interactive systems within larger systems (i.e., communities, nations) has exceeded measurement capabilities to a large degree. As a result, there has been a loss of clarity of the behavioral assessment enterprise.

Given the extensive comingling of assessment and treatment throughout the behavioral parent training process, clinicians and researchers face the real danger of becoming either overly restrictive in their adherence to the individual level of analysis or loosely organized around vague family systems treatment goals. Indeed, Yando and Zigler (1984) argued that the recent emphasis on family systems theory in assessing and treating children with severe handicaps is not without risk. In particular, the determination of a functional relationship between targeted problems and particular treatments suffers in a wholesale acceptance of this model *unless* evidence is available to provide empirical support for its use. At present, the empirical evidence is suggestive, but not conclusive.

The long term utility of systems models for intervening with parents of children with severe handicaps will depend on future research demonstrating the ability of these models to generate predictive and reliable assessment data that lead to specific treatments and positive outcomes at various levels of the family system. To achieve this goal clinicians and researchers will have to adopt a multilevel, multimethod framework for assessing behavioral parent training outcomes.

AN ASSESSMENT
FRAMEWORK

The adoption of a systems perspective necessitates assessment at several levels of the family system: individual, family, and community. The interdependent nature of components of systems requires special efforts in outcome measurement (Schwartz, 1982).

Although direct observation remains the mainstay of behavioral assessment, there is increasing interest in the use of multiple evaluation methods, including direct observation, rating scales, checklists, and structured interviews. Given the proposal that behavioral parent training emphasize interactions within the family, additional evaluation methods are not only appropriate, but also desirable. Indeed, Lamb (1978) noted that recognition of the sequence and timing of the behavior of participants is essential for investigating social interactions. Frequency counts, for example, would be poor dependent measures in certain cases because they do not yield interactional data.

To provide the breadth of data necessary for analysis of family interactional processes, it is necessary to adopt a multimethod approach to data collection. This approach allows the clinician and researcher access to behavioral sequences with little inference necessary (using direct observation and an interaction code), family perceptions of complex processes (e.g., cohesion) that resist arbitrary chunking of behavior into units of analysis (using well-standardized measures of family process), to more phenomenologically oriented data (gleaned from structured interviews). It is beyond the scope of this chapter to review these methods in detail; for that the reader is referred to other sources (Odom & Shuster, 1986; Simeonsson, 1986; Winton, 1986). We will mention, however, several instruments that can be used to measure the variables we have discussed.

At the individual level the clinician is concerned with the specific behavioral excesses, deficits, and skills of the child with a severe handicap (Evans, 1985). In addition, specific skills or issues of individual family members are evaluated. For example, it may be appropriate to evaluate a father's ability to deliver reinforcers contingently, as well as stress or potential psychopathology (using the Parenting Stress Index, Abidin, 1983; or the Minnesota Multiphasic Personality Inventory, respectively).

At the family level there are four areas of potential interest: family climate, family relationships, family structure, and the family life cycle. Family climate represents the psychological atmosphere present within the family. It is assumed that the psychological climate influences—and is influenced by—the behavior of family members. The Family Environment Scale (Moos & Moos, 1981) is one of the best known measures of family climate. Family relationships represent the quality of interactions between members of various family subsystems (e.g., marital, sibling, extended family). Appropriate measures might include the Locke-Wallace marital inventory (Locke & Wallace, 1959), The Parent-Child Interaction Scale (Farran, Comfort-Smith & Kasari, 1985) or the Family Perception Questionnaire (Harris, Handleman, & Palmer, 1985).

Family structure assessment involves a determination of the roles assumed by individual family members and the ways in which these roles coalesce to form the pattern of interaction unique to the particular family. For example, Harris (1982) describes the role of the "parentified sibling," one where an older child assumes parental responsibilities for the care of a brother or sister with a handicap. While such a role does not necessarily lead to a pathological family structure, to the extent that the normal development of the nonhandicapped sibling is affected it may well lead to an imbalanced family structure. Other structures to consider include the boundaries between the parental and sibling subsystems and the maintenance of a healthy relationship within the marital system. Minuchin (1974) offered extensive guidance on family structures and their assessment.

Much has been said about the importance of the family life cycle in the assessment and treatment process. It is essential to contextualize the child and family within the appropriate phase of the life cycle. Doing so allows the professional to predict stressors (e.g., the child's upcoming "aging out" of public educational services) and place parental distress or family upheaval within a normal developmental context, as appropriate. Turnbull and Winton (1984) describe 42 potential transitional stressors across the life cycle of the family with a severely handicapped member.

At the community level the clinician is concerned with such issues as availability of resources, insularity, and skills in networking and advocacy. Powers and Handleman (1984) described resources to assess with families, including human resources (e.g., availability of persons to participate in the intervention); technological resources (e.g., apparatus needed for treatment, specific competencies required of interveners); physical resources (e.g., the availability of community sites in which to conduct training); and financial resources (e.g., either personal funds or coverage from third party payors).

The isolation felt by many families who have children with severe handicaps is often a source of considerable pain. Wahler and Dumas (1984) offered extensive documentation of the effects of maternal insularity on parent-child interactions, arguing that, if left unattended, this variable may severely compromise behavioral treatment. Their work suggested that formal assessment of the frequency and quality of outside contacts with extended family, friends, or other community members be considered where such contact will be necessary for successful treatment outcomes (e.g., school placement). To the extent that parental isolation represents a clinical issue, it may become an adjunctive focus of parent training.

Parents are often expected to be the primary advocates for their children. Although some parents accept this role readily and acquire the required competencies quickly, for others advocacy and networking on behalf of their child with a severe handicap is superceded by priorities such as adequate shelter or food. Consideration of the family's ability to advocate effectively for their child or to access the community resources to fulfill that role is an important task for professionals to address.

CONCLUSION

The adoption of a systems perspective on behavioral parent training raises formidable challenges concerning issues of definition, measurement, the integration of data derived from molecular and molar levels of analysis, and the prediction of differential treatments given family developmental, interpersonal, and situational variables. Moreover, the integration of behavioral and systems theory models for purposes of assessing and treating families of children with severe handicaps represents a major shift in both the content and process of parent training. Much work remains to be done before we can feel entirely comfortable with the empirical foundation for integration. We know virtually nothing about the comparative effect of traditional behavioral parent training versus behavioral/systems parent training on generalization and maintenance of parent and child behavior changes or on family functioning. Indeed, the question of theoretical compatibility of behavioral and systems approaches remains largely undiscussed. On a more fundamental level, current models for data analysis in behavior therapy—which emphasize the evaluation of content and products—may be insufficient to measure treatment process, an integral index of change in family systems theory.

These issues, while daunting, should not obscure the fact that failures and incomplete successes are all too common in behavioral parent training. Clearly, the time for complacency has not yet arrived.

REFERENCES

Abidin, R. (1983). *Parenting Stress Index*. Charlottesville, VA: Pediatric Psychology Press.

Arnold, S., Sturgis, E., & Forehand, R. (1977). Training a parent to teach communication skills: A case study. *Behavior Modification, 1,* 259–276.

Baker, B. L., Heifetz, L. J., & Murphy, D. M. (1980). Behavioral training for parents of mentally retarded children: One year follow-up. *American Journal of Mental Deficiency, 87,* 31–38.

Barber, K., Barber, M., & Clark, H. B. (1983). Establishing a community oriented group home and ensuring its survival: A case study of failure. *Analysis and Intervention in Developmental Disabilities, 3,* 227–238.

Barbrack, C. R. (1985). Negative outcome in behavior therapy. In D. T. Mays & C. M. Franks (Eds.), *Negative outcome in psychotherapy and what to do about it* (pp. 76–105). New York: Springer.

Baum, C. G., & Forehand, R. (1981). Long-term follow-up assessment of parent training by use of multiple-outcome measures. *Behavior Therapy, 12,* 643–652.

Bernal, M. E., Klinnert, M.D., & Schultz, L. A. (1980). Outcome evaluation of behavioral parent training and client-centered parent counseling for children with conduct problems. *Journal of Applied Behavior Analysis, 13,* 677–691.

Bronfenbrenner, U. (1986). Ecology of the family as a context for human development. *Developmental Psychology, 22,* 723–742.

Christensen, A., Johnson, S. M., Phillips, S., & Glasgow, R. E. (1980). Cost effectiveness in behavioral family therapy. *Behavior Therapy, 11,* 208–226.

Dadds, M. R., Sanders, M. R., & James, J. E. (1987). The generalization of treatment effects in parent training with multidistressed parents. *Behavioural Psychotherapy, 15,* 289–313.

Dangle, R. F., & Polster, R. A. (1984). WINNING!: A systematic, empirical approach to parent training. In R. A. Polster & R. F. Dangle (Eds.), *Parent training: Foundations of research and practice* (pp. 162–201). New York: The Guilford Press.

Evans, I. M. (1985). Building systems models as a strategy for target behavior selection in clinical assessment. *Behavioral Assessment, 7,* 21–32.

Eyberg, S. M., & Matarazzo, R. G. (1980). Training parents as therapists: A comparison between individual parent-child interaction training and group didactic training. *Journal of Clinical Psychology, 36,* 492–499.

Farran, D., Comfort-Smith, M., & Kasari, C. (1985). *Factors affecting parent-child interactions with young handicapped children.* Paper presented at the meeting of the Society for Research on Child Development, Toronto.

Favell, S. E., & Reid, D. H. (1984). Group instruction for persons with severe disabilities: A critical review. *Journal of the Association for Persons with Severe Handicaps, 9,* 167–177.

Featherstone, H. (1980). *A difference in the family.* New York: Basic Books.

Forehand, R., & King, H. E. (1977). Noncompliant children: Effects of parent training on behavior and attitude change. *Behavior Modification, 1,* 93–109.

Forehand, R., Rogers, T., McMahon, R. J., Wells, K. C., & Griest, D. L. (1981). Teaching parents to modify child behavior problems: An examination of some follow-up data. *Journal of Pediatric Psychology, 6,* 313-322.

Forehand, R., Sturgis, E. T., McMahon, R. J., Aguar, D., Green, K., Wells, K. C., & Breiner, J. (1979). Parent behavioral training to modify child noncompliance: Treatment generalization across time and from home to school. *Behavior Modification, 3,* 3–25.

Fowler, S. A., Johnson, M. R., Whitman, T. L., & Zukotynski, G. (1978). Teaching a parent in the home to train self-help skills and increase compliance in her profoundly retarded adult daughter. *AAESPH Review, 3,* 151–161.

Friman, P. C., Barnard, J. D., Altman, K., & Wolf, M. M. (1986). Parent and teacher use of DRO and DRI to reduce aggressive behavior. *Analysis and Intervention in Developmental Disabilities, 6,* 319–330.

Griest, D. L., & Forehand, R. (1982). How can I get any parent training done with all these other problems going on? The role of family variables in child behavior therapy. *Child and Family Behavior Therapy, 4,* 73–80.

Griest, D. L., Forehand, R., & Wells, K. C. (1981). Follow-up assessment of parent behavioral training: An analysis of who will participate. *Child Study Journal, 11,* 221–229.

Hall, R. V., Christler, C., Cranston, S., & Tucker, B. (1970). Teachers and parents as researchers using multiple-baseline tactics. *Journal of Applied Behavior Analysis, 4,* 247–255.

Harris, S. L. (1982). A family systems approach to behavioral training with parents of autistic children. *Child and Family Behavior Therapy, 4,* 21–35.

Harris, S. L. (1983). *Families of the developmentally disabled: A guide to behavioral intervention.* Elmsford, NY: Pergamon.

Harris, S. L. (1984). Intervention planning for the family of the autistic child: A multilevel assessment of the family system. *Journal of Marital and Family Therapy, 10,* 157–166.

Harris, S. L., (1986). Parents as teachers: A four to seven year follow up of parents of children with autism. *Child and Family Behavior Therapy, 8,* 39–47.

Harris, S. L. (1988). Parent training: An ecological/systems perspective. In M. D. Powers (Ed.), *Expanding systems of service delivery for persons with developmental disabilities* (pp. 53–65). Baltimore: Paul H. Brookes.

Harris, S. L., Handleman, J. S., & Palmer, C. (1985). Parents and grandparents view the autistic child. *Journal of Autism and Developmental Disorders, 15,* 127–137.

Harris, S. L., & Powers, M. D. (1984). Behavior therapists look at the impact of the autistic child on the family system. In E. Schopler & G. B. Mesibov (Eds.), *The effects of autism on the family* (pp. 207–224). New York: Plenum.

Harris, S. L., Wolchik, S. A., & Milch, R. E. (1983). Changing the speech of autistic children and their parents. *Child and Family Behavior Therapy, 4,* 151–173.

Harris, S. L., Wolchik, S. A., & Weitz, S. (1981). The acquisition of language skills by autistic children: Can parents do the job? *Journal of Autism and Developmental Disorders, 11,* 373–384.

Heifetz, L. J. (1977). Behavioral training for parents of retarded children. *American Journal of Mental Deficiency, 82,* 194–203.

Holmes, N., Hemsley, R., Rickett, J., & Likierman, H. (1982). Parents as cotherapists: Their perceptions of a home-based behavioral treatment for autistic children. *Journal of Autism and Developmental Disorders, 12,* 331–342.

Holroyd, J., & McArthur, D. (1976). Mental retardation and stress of the parents: A contrast between Down's syndrome and childhood autism. *American Journal of Mental Deficiency, 80,* 431–436.

Kaiser, A. P., & Fox, J. J. (1986). Behavioral parent training research: Contributions to an ecological analysis of families of handicapped children. In J. J. Gallagher & P. M. Vietze (Eds.), *Families of handicapped persons: Research, programs and policy issues.* Baltimore: Paul H. Brookes.

Kelly, M. L., Embry, L. H., & Baer, D. M. (1979). Skills for child management and family support. *Behavior Modification, 3,* 373–396.

Kleinman, A. M., Eisenberg, L., & Good, B. (1978). Culture, illness, and care: Clinical lessons from anthropologic and cross-cultural research. *Annals of Internal Medicine, 88,* 251–258.

Koegel, R. L., Glahn, T. J., & Nieminen, G. S. (1978). Generalization of parent-training results. *Journal of Applied Behavior Analysis, 11,* 95–109.

Koegel, R. L., Schreibman, L., Johnson, J., O'Neill, R. E., & Dunlap, G. (1984). Collateral effects of parent training on families with autistic children. In R. F. Dangel and R. N. Polster (Eds.), *Parent-training: Foundations of research and practice.* New York: Guilford Press.

Kovitz, K. E. (1976). Comparing group and individual methods for training parents in child management techniques. In E. J. Mash, L. C. Handy, & L. A. Hamerlynck (Eds.), *Behavior modification approaches to parenting* (pp. 124–140). New York: Brunner/Mazel.

Lamb, M. (1978). Influence of the child on marital quality and family interaction during the prenatal, perinatal, and infancy periods. In R. Lerner & G. Spanier (Eds.), *Child influences on marital and family interaction: A life-span perspective* (pp. 137–163). New York: Academic Press.

Lobato, D., & Barrera, R. (1988). Impact of siblings on children with handicaps. In M. D. Powers (Ed.), *Expanding systems of service delivery for persons with developmental disabilities.* (pp. 43–52). Baltimore: Paul H. Brookes.

Locke, H. J., & Wallace, K. M. (1959). Short marital adjustment and prediction tests: Their reliability and validity. *Marriage and Family Living, 21,* 251–255.

Lovaas, O. I., Koegel, R. L., Simmons, J. Q., & Long, J. S. (1973). Some generalizations and follow-up measures and autistic children in behavior therapy. *Journal of Applied Behavior Analysis, 6,* 131–161.

Lutzker, J. R., McGimsey, J. F., McRae, S., & Campbell, R. V. (1983). Behavior parent training: There's so much more to do. *The Behavior Therapist, 6,* 110–112.

Mash, E. J. (1984). Families with problem children. In A. Doyle, D. Gold, & D. Moskowitz (Eds.), *Children in families with stress* (pp. 65–84). Behavioral assessment of child and family disorders: Contemporary approaches. *Behavioral Assessment, 9,* 201–205.

McMahon, R. J., Forehand, R., Griest, D. L., & Wells, K. C. (1981). Who drops out of treatment during parent behavioral training? *Behavioral Counseling Quarterly, 1,* 79–85.

Mesibov, G. B. (1983). Current perspectives and issues in autism and adolescence. In E. Schopler & G. B. Mesibov (Eds.), *Autism in adolescents and adults* (pp. 37–53). New York: Plenum.

Miller, J. S. (1978). *Living systems.* New York: McGraw-Hill.

Minuchin, S. (1974). *Families and family therapy.* Cambridge, MA: Harvard University Press.

Moos, R. H. (1979). Improving social settings by social climate and feedback. In R. Munoz, L. Snowden, & J. Kelly (Eds.), *Social and psychological research in community settings.* San Francisco: Jossey-Bass.

Moos, R. H., & Moos, B. S. (1981). *Family environment scale.* Palo Alto, CA: Consulting Psychologists Press.

Neef, N. A., Shafer, M. S., Egel, A. L., Cataldo, M. F., & Parrish, J. M. (1983). The class specific effects of compliance training with "Do" and "Don't" requests. *Journal of Applied Behavior Analysis, 16,* 81–99.

Nordquist, V. M. (1971). The modification of a child's enuresis: Some response-response relationships. *Journal of Applied Behavior Analysis, 4,* 241–247.

O'Dell, S. L. (1985). Progress in parent training. In M. Herson, R. Eisler, & P. Miller (Eds.), *Progress in behavior modification, Vol. 19* (pp. 57–108). New York: Academic Press, Inc.

O'Dell, S. L., Krug, W. W., O'Quin, J. A., & Kasnetz, M. (1980). Media-assisted parent training—A further analysis. *The Behavior Therapist, 3,* 19–21.

O'Dell, S. L., Krug, W. W., Patterson, J. N., & Faustman, W. O. (1980). An assessment of methods for training parents in the use of time-out. *Journal of Behavior Therapy and Experimental Psychiatry, 11,* 21–25.

O'Dell, S. L., Mahoney, N., Horton, W., & Turner, P. (1979). Media-assisted parent training: Alternative models. *Behavior Therapy, 16,* 103–110.

O'Dell, S. L., O'Quin, J. A., Alford, B. A., O'Briant, A. L., Bradlyn, A. S., Giebenhain, J. E. (1982). Predicting the acquisition of parenting skills via four training methods. *Behavior Therapy, 13,* 194–208.

Odom, S. L., & Shuster, S. K. (1986). Naturalistic inquiry and the assessment of young handicapped children and their families. *Topics of Early Childhood Special Education, 6,* 68–82.

Patterson, G. R., & Fleishman, M. J. (1979). Maintenance of treatment effects: Some considerations concerning family systems and follow-up data. *Behavior Therapy, 10,* 168–185.

Patterson, G. R., & Reid, J. B. (1973). Intervention for families of aggressive boys: A replication study. *Behaviour Research and Therapy, 11,* 383–394.

Peed, S., Roberts, M., & Forehand, R. (1977). Evaluation of the effectiveness of a standardized parent training program in altering the interaction of mothers and their noncompliant children. *Behavior Modification, 1,* 323–350.

Polster, R. A., & Dangle, R. F. (1984). *Parent training: Foundations of research and practice.* New York: Guilford Press.

Powers, M. D. (1986a). Consultation and counseling with families of young children with severe handicaps. In M. K. Hawryluk (chair), *Family involvement in early childhood special education: School psychology perspectives.* Symposium presented at the 94th annual convention of the American Psychological Association, Washington, D.C.

Powers, M. D. (1986b). Promoting community-based services: Implication for program design, implementation, and public policy. *Journal of the Association for Persons with Severe Handicaps, 11,* 309–315.

Powers, M. D., (1988). A systems approach to serving persons with severe developmental disabilities. In M. D. Powers (Ed.), *Expanding systems of service delivery for persons with developmental disabilities* (pp. 1–14). Baltimore: Paul H. Brookes.

Powers, M. D., & Bruey, C. T. (1988). Treating the family system. In M. D. Powers (Ed.), *Expanding systems of service delivery for persons with developmental disabilities* (pp. 17–41). Baltimore: Paul H. Brookes.

Powers, M. D., & Handleman, J. S. (1984). *Behavioral assessment of severe developmental disabilities.* Rockville, MD: Aspen Press.

Reppucci, N. D., & Saunders, J. T. (1983). Focal issues for institutional change. *Professional Psychology: Research and Practice, 14,* 514–528.

Rios, J. D., & Gutierrez, J. M. (1986). Parent training with non-traditional families: An unresolved issue. *Child and Family Behavior Therapy, 7,* 33–45.

Rosenberg, M. S., Reppucci, N. D., & Linney, J. A. (1983). Issues in the implementation of human service programs: Examples from a parent training project for high-risk families. *Analysis and Intervention in Developmental Disabilities, 3,* 215–225.

Russo, D. C., Cataldo, M. F., & Cushing, P. J. (1981). Compliance training and behavioral covariation in the treatment of multiple behavior problems. *Journal of Applied Behavior Analysis, 14,* 209–222.

Schreibman, L., Koegel, R. L., Mills, D. L., & Burke, J. C. (1984). Training parent-child interactions. In E. Schopler & G. B. Mesibov (Eds.), *The effects of autism on the family* (pp. 187–205). New York: Plenum.

Schwartz, G. E. (1982). Integrating psychobiology and behavior therapy: A systems perspective. In G. T. Wilson & C. M. Franks (Eds.), *Contemporary behavior therapy* (pp. 119–141). New York: Guilford Press.

Simeonsson, R. J. (1986). *Psychological and developmental assessment of special children.* Newton, MA: Allyn & Bacon.

Snell, M. E., & Beckman-Brindley, S. (1984). Family involvement in intervention with children having severe handicaps. *Journal of the Association for Persons with Severe Handicaps, 9,* 213–230.

Speck, R., & Attneave, C. L. (1973). *Family networks: Retribalization and healing.* New York: Pantheon.

Strain, P. S., Young, C., & Horowitz, J. (1981). Generalized behavior change during oppositional child training: An examination of child and family demographic variables. *Behavior Modification, 5,* 15–26.

Turnbull, A. Brotherson, M., & Summers, J. (1986). The impact of deinstitutionalization on families: A family systems approach. In R. Bruinicks (Ed.), *Living and learning in the least restrictive environment* (pp. 26–52). Baltimore: Paul H. Brookes.

Turnbull, A., & Winton, P. (1984). Parent involvement policy and practice: Current research and implications for families with young, severely handicapped children. In J. Blacher (Ed.), *Severely handicapped young children and their families: Research in review* (pp. 377–397). New York: Academic Press.

Voeltz, L. M., & Evans, I. M. (1982). The assessment of behavioral interrelationships in child behavior therapy. *Behavioral Assessment, 4,* 131–165.

von Bertalanffy, L. V. (1968). *General systems theory.* New York: George Braziller.

Wahler, R. G. (1980). The insular mother: Her problems in parent-child treatment. *Journal of Applied Behavior Analysis, 13,* 207–219.

Wahler, R. G., & Afton, A. D. (1980). Attentional processes in insular and noninsular mothers: Some differences in their summary reports about child problem behavior. *Child Behavior Therapy, 2,* 25–42.

Wahler, R. G., & Dumas, J. E. (1984). Changing the observational coding styles of insular and noninsular mothers: A step toward maintenance of parent training effects. In R. F. Dangel & R. A. Polster (Eds.), *Parent training: Foundations of research and practice* (pp. 379–416). New York: Guilford Press.

Webster-Stratton, C. (1985). Predictors of treatment outcome in parent training for conduct disordered children. *Behavior Therapy, 16,* 223–243.

Winton, P. (1986). The developmentally delayed child within the family context. In *Advances in special education* Vol. 5, (pp. 219–255). Greenwich, CT: JAI Press.

Yando, R., & Zigler, E. (1984). Severely handicapped children and their families: A synthesis. In J. Blacher (Ed.), *Severely handicapped children and their families: Research in review* (pp. 401–416). New York: Academic Press.

Treating Aberrant Behavior Through Effective Staff Management
A Developing Technology

Dennis H. Reid,
Marsha B. Parsons,
and
Carolyn W. Green
Western Carolina Center, Morganton, NC

An area warranting serious concern in the design and implementation of treatment programs for aberrant behavior among persons who have developmental disabilities is the effective management of residential staff performance. A primary reason for such concern is the recognition that residential staff are frequently required to serve a client population that exhibits an increased incidence of severe behavior disorders relative to previous institutional populations (Reid & Schepis, 1986). In addition, it has become apparent that the existence of an effective technology for treating aberrant behavior as represented in the professional literature (see earlier chapters in this monograph) will actually benefit few clients if caregivers do not proficiently *apply* the technology (Stolz, 1981). It has also become apparent that, generally, the type of residential staff performance necessary to consistently provide therapeutic client services—including services necessary for treating behavior disorders—will not occur without an effective managerial process (Favell, Favell, Riddle, & Risley, 1984). If effective management practices do not exist in residential settings, then staff performance often not only represents less than optimal application of behavioral treatment strategies, but also can actually foster the development and/or continuance of aberrant client behavior (Reid & Schepis, 1986).

The reasons for the difficulties in ensuring proficient staff performance in the provision of residential client services have been thoroughly discussed. To summarize, two primary reasons seem to be that, in general, (a) institutional staff such as direct care personnel typically have had little or no formal training before assuming their caregiving and treatment roles (Burch, Reiss, & Bailey, 1987; Zlomke & Benjamin, 1983) and (b) such staff are faced with a difficult task that often must be completed with limited resources (Reid & Shoemaker, 1984). Nevertheless, it is essential that caregivers be assisted to overcome such obstacles if treatment programs for aberrant behavior among residential clients are to be effective. The effectiveness of treatment programs is particularly dependent on the competent performance of direct care personnel because these staff generally spend the most time with, and have the greatest impact on, clients in residential facilities who manifest the behavior disorders (Bensberg & Barnett, 1966).

As alluded to earlier, the responsibility for ensuring that the performance of direct care staff reflects appropriate service provision in essence falls on the managers or supervisors in residential facilities. In order to fulfill such a responsibility, managers must of course know how to ensure that their staff supervisees are performing their job duties appropriately; the managers must have the knowledge and skills to effectively manage the work performance of their staff. Unfortunately, many if not most human service managers enter their managerial roles without any preparation to be managers; most managers were formerly trained as human service clinicians (psychologists, teachers, etc.). Consequently, many managers in residential settings do not have the necessary skills and knowledge to effectively manage the performance of direct care personnel in terms of ensuring satisfactory performance.

Recently, applied behavioral researchers have begun to develop a technology to assist managers in their task of supervising staff performance. The development of a staff management technology has been the focus of investigators within the growing field of organizational behavior management, which involves the systematic application of principles of behavior change to staff performance in the work place (see *Journal of Organizational Behavior Management*, Volumes 1–8). This approach to staff management is built upon the ongoing development of effective procedures for improving staff performance based on the results of applied behavioral research in work settings and, of special concern here, including residential agencies for persons who have developmental disabilities and who exhibit behavior disorders. It is the purpose of this chapter to describe the developing technology of organizational behavior management for managing residential staff performance.

The chapter consists of five main sections. In the first four sections, the component steps of organizational behavior management (Reid & Shoemaker, 1984) are described, along with the applied research that focuses on the importance and/or efficacy of each step in regard to improving staff performance. The fifth section summarizes the overall state of the existing technology of staff management, as well as areas that warrant the attention of applied researchers for continued development and refinement of the technology.

COMPONENT STEPS OF
BEHAVIORAL STAFF
MANAGEMENT: SUMMARY
AND RESEARCH
OUTCOMES

Defining Performance Responsibilities

The first component step in organizational behavior management involves behaviorally defining staff performance responsibilities. The purpose of this step is to describe clearly *what* a staff person is expected to do as part of a job, as well as to delineate the performance parameters of the job in terms of *where, when,* and often with *whom* (i.e., which residents) the specific performance should occur (Reid & Whitman, 1983). For example, if direct care staff are to effectively implement a time-out procedure to reduce a given resident's aggressive behavior (Katz & Lutzker, 1980), the staff must know exactly what resident behaviors should result in time-out, how long the time-out procedure should be implemented, where time-out should occur across different locations in which the resident may be, and so on. By very clearly defining what a staff person is expected to do, the likelihood of the staff member knowing and understanding what is expected of him/her increases. Additionally, well-defined job responsibilities facilitate a manager's task of monitoring staff performance (see next section) in that it is easier to determine whether or not given duties are being completed by staff in an acceptable manner. In this regard, the primary purpose of this first step in organizational behavior management is really to set the occasion for implementing subsequent supervisory procedures to actually change respective staff performances rather than to alter ongoing work behavior per se; however, in some cases behaviorally specifying staff job responsibilities can have the effect of improving day-to-day work performance (Iwata, Bailey, Brown, Foshee, & Alpern, 1976; Sneed & Bible, 1979). In and of itself, though, performance specification should not be heavily relied on as a procedure to change routine job behavior; such a process does not *consistently* result in significant changes in performance (Quilitch, 1975; Seys & Duker, 1978).

Monitoring Staff Performance

The second component step in organizational behavior management is supervisory monitoring of specified staff performances. Once performance responsibilities have been clearly specified (first step), a supervisor or his/her designee must then observe staff performance in a frequent and systematic manner to determine whether staff are appropriately fulfilling their identified responsibilities. The primary goal of this step is to obtain an objective and representative record of what staff are doing. For example, systematic monitoring of staffs' implementation of punishment procedures with client behavior disorders is usually necessary in order to help ensure that the procedures are being applied consistently, effectively, and safely (Repp & Deitz, 1978). Information resulting from a monitoring system allows a supervisor to determine accurately what (if any) additional managerial actions are necessary to alter inadequate performance or to maintain satisfactory performance.

One of the major advantages of systematic monitoring systems is that the availability of data-based, representative indices of the adequacy of staff performance sets the occasion for an objective and fair managerial process with staff. Without such systems, managers are typically left with only their subjective opinions of the performance adequacy or inadequacy of staff and/or similar opinions of other agency personnel, a process that can lead to numerous difficulties ranging from performance evaluation disagreements between supervisors and supervisees to (unintentionally) biased decision making on the part of managers. A number of monitoring systems have been developed that can be used as part of residential operations to obtain objective information on staff performance, including performance checklist observations (Burch et al., 1987), momentary time sampling procedures (Seys & Duker, 1986), interval observation processes (Page, Iwata, & Reid, 1982) and permanent product monitoring (Ivancic, Reid, Iwata, Faw, & Page, 1981). Although each of these types of monitoring systems has its own advantages and disadvantages in regard to its general utility (the interested reader is referred to the respective references for additional information), each has been successfully used in organizational behavior management applications in residential settings.

In some ways, it seems logical that the effects of systematic monitoring of staff performance would be similar to the (intermittent) effects of performance specification just noted in that the monitoring would have an actual behavior change impact on what staff are doing. That is, staff would seem to be more likely to perform a given job task if they know what to do *and* that their supervisor will be routinely observing their performance. Currently though, available research data—albeit a limited amount at this point—do not support the view that systematic staff monitoring systems result in significant changes in daily job performance of staff (Hagen, Craighead, & Paul, 1975; Ivancic et al., 1981). In terms of what can be concluded with any scientific verification, performance monitoring generally should be considered in the same manner as performance specification:

an important and necessary component of an overall organizational behavior management approach, but not a performance change step per se.

Although typical staff monitoring systems to date have not been shown to impact staff performance when used without other components of organizational behavior management approaches, there are two somewhat specialized types of monitoring processes that seem more likely to affect staff behavior in this regard. The first of these is *staff self-monitoring*. Some preliminary research findings suggest that if staff monitor and maintain records on specified areas of their own work behavior, such performance areas are likely to be beneficially affected in regard to increasing and/or maintaining their appropriate occurrence (Burg, Reid, & Lattimore, 1979; Kissel, Whitman, & Reid, 1983; Seys & Duker, 1978). Continued research is needed to determine more conclusively the potential behavior change effects of staff self-monitoring.

The second type of monitoring that seems likely to affect behavior change with staff is an *external monitoring process* as used by governmental regulatory agencies such as the federal Health Care Finance Administration's surveys of agency compliance with the Title XIX Medicaid Program for Intermediate Care Facilities for the Mentally Retarded. This type of monitoring is external in that personnel who are not employed by a given human service agency conduct the observations within the agency in contrast to the more routine, internal systems in which personnel indigenous to an agency conduct the monitoring. Generally, external monitoring processes used by regulatory agencies are characterized by their overtness (it is quite apparent when observations are occurring) as well as by their relative infrequency (they typically occur no more than once or twice per year). Most likely because of these features, and the fact that the results of the monitoring often have a potentially serious impact on a human service agency—such as loss of government funding—staff tend to respond differently during an external agency review relative to routine work performance, and generally more desirably from a client service standpoint. However, whatever improvements occur as a result of these types of monitoring systems seem to be shortlived (Quilitch, de Longchamps, Warden, & Szczepaniak, 1977) and there is no hard evidence to suggest that such monitoring systems significantly affect day-to-day staff performance in a manner that would beneficially impact client service provision (Repp & Barton, 1980).

Teaching New Skills to Staff

The third step in organizational behavior management is staff training: teaching new work skills to staff. This component step represents a procedure that is frequently recommended for resolving performance problems of direct care staff (Bensberg & Barnett, 1966; Gardner, 1973). Indeed, given the typical lack of preparation for their caregiver roles as noted earlier and some of the rather complex treatment procedures that they are expected to implement with clients who have behavior problems, direct care personnel usually do need to be trained to perform certain tasks once they begin employment in a residential facility. In addition, even well-trained and experienced staff frequently require periodic training to improve given performance duties because the services they are expected to provide often change as, for example, new and revised treatment strategies for aberrant client behavior are developed. Such a need for training is particularly important in regard to treatment of client behavior disorders if human service agencies are to continuously upgrade their treatment programs to coincide with new treatment developments that result from research on aberrant behavior.

Although staff training is often quite important for the reasons just noted, the utility of this component step for changing day-to-day staff performance in the workplace is frequently exaggerated. Staff training programs are often conducted within typical residential facilities in an attempt to resolve problematic staff performances despite the existence of a considerable amount of applied research data documenting that staff training in and of itself will not resolve the situations (Greene, Willis, Levy, & Bailey, 1978; Montegar, Reid, Madsen, & Ewell, 1977; Quilitch, 1975). To illustrate, many staff performance problems exist not because staff do not possess the necessary work skills, but because they do not apply these work skills in the daily work routine (Greene et al., 1978; Montegar et al., 1977). In such situations staff training programs essentially amount to attempting to teach the staff to do something they already know how to do, and have no real impact on work performance. Also, in a number of cases in which performance problems actually are attributable (at least in part) to lack of necessary work skills among staff, staff training programs do not resolve the problems because of a lack of skill carryover: that is, although staff may learn appropriate work skills as a result of a staff training program, they still do not consistently apply the skills during the routine workday (Whitman, Scibak, & Reid, 1983). The reasons for the lack of skill carryover, the methods of enhancing routine application of newly acquired work skills, will be noted later in this chapter. Suffice it to say at this point that it has become quite clear from a considerable amount of research on staff behavior in residential facilities that staff training endeavors should be considered as a step that is *often necessary* for improving day-to-day staff performance but *rarely sufficient* in this regard.

When staff training endeavors are needed to assist in improving staff performance (i.e., when performance problems exist at least somewhat because of a lack of relevant work skills among staff), a variety of procedures are available for conducting the training. Training programs can include, for example, verbal (Quilitch, 1975) and/or written instructions (Page, Christian, Iwata, Reid, Crow, & Dorsey, 1981) presented in individual (van den Pol, Reid, & Fuqua, 1983) and/or group (Fitzgerald, Reid, Schepes, Faw, Welty, & Pyfer, 1984) formats, pictorial instruction (Fielding, Errickson, & Bettin, 1971; Stoddard, McIlvane, McDonagh, & Kledaras, 1986), performance demonstrations through live modeling (Gladstone & Spencer, 1977; Ivancic et al., 1981; Mansdorf & Burstein, 1986) or videotape presentation (Kissel et al., 1983), performance practice (Faw, Reid, Schepis, Fitzgerald, & Welty, 1981) including role playing (Adams, Tallon, & Rimell, 1980; Gardner, 1972) and/or verbal rehearsal (Stoddard et al., 1986), and various types of programmed instruction presentations (Ford, 1983). Each of these procedures represents an *antecedent* approach to staff training in terms of instructing staff in how to perform a new work skill before or during the time staff actually exhibit the performance (Whitman et al., 1983).

Because each antecedent procedure has its own idiosyncratic advantages and disadvantages, space limitations prohibit a discussion of the relative benefits of each strategy here (for elaboration, see Gardner, 1973; Miller & Lewin, 1980; Reid & Green, in press). However, overall, antecedent procedures are not consistently effective in teaching proficient application of new skills unless they are used in conjunction with *consequence* procedures that provide staff with explicit positive or negative outcomes regarding their performance proficiency once the staff attempt to apply the skills targeted in the training program (Whitman et al., 1983).

A variety of consequence procedures have been used in staff training programs in residential facilities, with the vast majority involving some type of performance feedback (Ford, 1980). Feedback as part of training programs regarding staff's proficiency or nonproficiency in applying new work skills has been presented verbally to staff (Fabry & Reid, 1978; Gardner, 1972; Reid, Parsons, McCarn, Green, Phillips, & Schepis, 1985), in writing to individual staff persons (Shoemaker & Reid, 1980), in writing via public display for groups of staff (Greene et al., 1978; Ivancic et al., 1981), through videotaped replay (Kissel et al., 1983), and by way of staff self-recording feedback on their own performance (Korabek, Reid, & Ivancic, 1981). As with the various types of antecedent training strategies, each of the consequence procedures typically has its own relative strengths and weaknesses (for discussion, see Gardner, 1973; Reid & Green, in press).

The treatment of choice regarding the specific staff training procedure that is likely to be most effective depends on a variety of factors associated with the particular situation in which a job skill is to be trained and applied. Such factors include, for example, the type of skill to be taught, ranging from a complex skill that is used infrequently such as intervening during a client's aggressive physical attack (van den Pol et al., 1983) to a relatively simple skill that is used repetitively such as providing a praise statement for appropriate client behavior (Gladstone & Spencer, 1977). In addition, the resources available for training must be considered, such as readily accessible equipment (e.g., computers) (Smith & Wells, 1983), as well as the amount of prior training and/or background of the staff trainees (Page et al., 1981). However, there are also several characteristics that seem to be germane to any effective staff training program. First, combinations of procedures within a multifaceted program are more likely to be effective than is reliance on one training procedure used in isolation (Ivancic et al., 1981). Second, generally, the more similar the staff training environment and conditions are to the actual work situation in which staff are routinely expected to use the skills, the more beneficial the training program is likely to be (Lattimore, Stephens, Favell, & Risley, 1984). The importance of making the training process as similar as possible to the normal work routine of staff is particularly relevant in regard to resolving the problem of lack of carryover of staff skills noted earlier. Third, it is crucial that the final phases of the training program include staffs' independent demonstration of the accurate implementation of the targeted skill (Reid & Green, in press). Finally, it is paramount that the staff training program be followed by an active management component to support staffs' use of the newly acquired skill within the day-to-day work environment (see next section).

As implied in the preceding paragraphs, there has been a rather substantial amount of applied behavioral research on methods of training mental retardation staff. Of particular interest here, however, is the research on training staff specifically to treat or manage client behavior problems. Although the importance of staff training components within treatment plans for client behavior disorders has been well noted (Repp & Deitz, 1978), there has been a relative dearth of research attention given to methods of conducting such training. The staff training research has heavily emphasized training staff in methods of developing adaptive behavior with clients in contrast to methods of decreasing maladaptive behaviors (Reid & Green, in press). Where research has targeted staff training endeavors in regard to decelerating behavior problems, the analogue nature of the research (van den Pol et al., 1983) and/or lack of valid experimental designs (Katz & Lutzker, 1980) have limited the conclusions that can be drawn from the research. Hence, a useful line of research involving mental retardation staff would be the demonstration of effective (and efficient) methods of training such staff to proficiently implement treatment programs for aberrant client behavior.

Changing and Managing Ongoing Performance

As suggested in the preceding sections, the primary function of the component steps discussed to this point is to set the occasion for taking specific managerial action to significantly change day-to-day staff performance. Changing ongoing staff performance within the routine worksite represents the fourth component step in organizational behavior management. This step, which represents the real essence of behavioral approaches to staff management, focuses on the systematic application of consequences for staff performance (Whitman et al., 1983).

The most frequently investigated type of consequence procedure in staff management has been performance feedback, through which a supervisor or other authority figure provides evaluative information to staff regarding their day-to-day work performance (Kreitner, Reif, & Morris, 1977; Panyan, Boozer, & Morris, 1970). Similar to the use of feedback in staff training programs as discussed earlier, a wide variety of feedback procedures have been used to improve onsite work performance (Ford, 1980). Feedback strategies have also been used to improve a wide variety of different types of job performances of residential staff. To illustrate, publicly posted feedback has been used effectively to increase the frequency of staff's implementation of assigned training programs with clients (Greene et al., 1978; Welsch, Ludwig, Radiker, & Krapfl, 1973), as well as staffs' timeliness in performing interdisciplinary team functions (Hutchison, Jarman, & Bailey, 1980) and communicating with administrative personnel (Quilitch, 1978). Verbal feedback has successfully increased social interactions between staff and clients (Brown, Willis, & Reid, 1981; Montegar et al., 1977) and individual, privately written feedback has improved administrative recordkeeping performances of staff (Repp & Deitz, 1979). Overall, results of the research on the use of feedback as just exemplified provide strong support for the efficacy of this consequence procedure in terms of improving residential staff performance, although more research is needed to determine the relative advantages of different types of feedback strategies (Balcazar, Hopkins, & Suarex, 1986; Reid & Whitman, 1983).

In essence, any consequence procedure involves at least a degree of performance feedback. However, there have also been a number of consequence applications used with residential staff that did not focus on feedback per se. Rather, the procedures were intended to reinforce appropriate staff performance by providing presumably desired events, items, privileges, or special recognition contingent on some commendable work behavior of staff. A wide variety of consequences have functioned to increase certain staff performances including, for example, bonus money (Pomerleau, Bobrove, & Smith, 1973; Pommer & Streedbeck, 1974; Realon, Wheeler, Spring, & Springer, 1986), preferred work schedules such as an increased number of days off on weekends (Iwata et al., 1976; Reid, Schuh-Wear, & Brannon, 1978), relief from certain work duties and/or assignment of preferred work tasks (Seys & Duker, 1978; Shoemaker & Reid, 1980), and commercial trading stamps (Bricker, Morgan, & Grabowski, 1972; Hollander & Plutchik, 1972; Hollander, Plutchik, & Horner, 1973). Although nonfeedback consequence procedures as just illustrated have been used successfully in organizational behavior management research, there are some serious disadvantages when considering use of the procedures as part of supervisory approaches in typical residential settings relative to more explicit performance feedback strategies (Wallace, Davis, Liberman, & Baker, 1973). Most apparently, some of the consequences can be expensive (e.g., trading stamps, money) for human service agencies and managers. Even if the consequences are not necessarily expensive, though, they often are somewhat effortful for managers to provide over extended time periods (e.g., rearranging staff work schedules). Management procedures that are costly and/or effortful for supervisors frequently have a rather low probability of being consistently used by managers, especially over long periods of time. In contrast, performance feedback procedures usually do not involve significant expense and are generally readily available for use by supervisors.

THE CURRENT STATE OF BEHAVIORAL STAFF MANAGEMENT: CONTRIBUTIONS AND RESEARCH GAPS

Currently, well over 50 investigations have demonstrated the effectiveness of organizational behavior management procedures for improving residential staff performance. A number of the investigations have also shown that as staff performance improved, there were increases in adaptive behavior among institutionalized persons who have developmental disabilities (Burgio, Whitman, & Reid, 1983; Greene et al., 1978) and, of particular interest for this monograph, decreases in aberrant behavior (Burg et al., 1979; Horner, 1980; Spangler & Marshall, 1983). The amount of the management research in this regard and the rather consistently demonstrated improvements in staff performance leave little doubt that organizational behavior management procedures represent very useful tools for residential managers and supervisors. However, the behavioral technology for managing staff performance is by no means complete and considerably more applied research is needed if residential managers are to be fully equipped to fulfill their task of ensuring satisfactory performances of their staff. In this regard, staff management research has been especially criticized for being limited in scope from two perspectives: (a) relatively restricted areas of staff performance have been targeted within given investigations (Christian, 1983; Frederiksen, 1984; Mayhew, Enyart, & Cone, 1979) and (b) the durability of changes in staff performance over time has not been consistently evaluated (Ivancic et al., 1981; Kunz et al., 1982).

Concern over the restricted focus of research on staff behavior centers on the inclusion of only one or a small number of staff performance areas within staff investigations as well as a focus on performance responsibilities that encompasses only a small amount of time. Generally, residential staff have a number of varying tasks to perform throughout the workday and it is not clear that impacting a small subset of those responsibilities during a 1- or 2-hour period through use of an organizational behavior management procedure represents a significant outcome. Because of this feature of most of the investigations to date on staff behavior, conclusions regarding the efficacy of behavioral staff management approaches for substantially improving comprehensive areas of residential staff performance cannot be drawn. Recently, though, researchers have begun to evaluate more comprehensive, wide scale applications of organizational behavior management procedures (Dyer, Schwartz, & Luce, 1984; Parsons, Schepis, Reid, McCarn, & Green, 1987; Prue, Krapful, Noah, Cannon, & Maley, 1980). The results of these investigations, along with the comprehensive and successful applications of behavioral staff management procedures in nonhuman service industries (Fox, Hopkins, & Anger, 1987), offer encouragement for the potential wide scale efficacy and applicability of such approaches for improving residential staff performance. Investigations that continue to expand the scope of organizational behavior management would be useful to determine the degree to which behavioral procedures can be used effectively and practically throughout an agency's managerial functioning.

The second primary concern with the staff research, that of the lack of evaluation of maintenance of initial changes in staff behavior accompanying a behavioral management intervention, is now beginning to be well addressed in the applied research literature. To illustrate, an earlier review of the organizational behavior management research in mental retardation settings indicated that among the few studies (less than one-third of all staff investigations) that reported follow-up data, evaluation periods averaged approximately 6 weeks, with only two studies reporting data for periods of more than 10 weeks (Reid & Whitman, 1983). In contrast, more recent investigations have included rather lengthy follow-up periods including, for example 5 months (Dyer et al., 1984), 7 months (Alavosius & Sulzer-Azaroff, 1986), and 2 years (Parsons et al., 1987) duration. Results of the latter investigations have suggested that behavioral management procedures can indeed be used both to improve residential staff performance and to *maintain* those improvements.

Several earlier reviews and/or discussions of the organizational behavior management research have also indicated areas warranting research in addition to the two primary areas just noted. Such areas include evaluating (and/or improving) the acceptability of behavioral management procedures among staff supervisors (Bernstein & Karan, 1978), more clearly defining the utility or nonutility of punishment procedures for improving staff performance (Balcazar et al., 1986), and determining the existing contingencies operating on staff performance in typical residential environments that lead to relatively common performance problems (Reid & Whitman, 1983). We agree in noting that each of these areas continues to warrant the attention of researchers. However, we would add to the recommended directions for applied research in organizational behavior management by asserting that (a) the primary components of an effective technology for improving and managing residential staff performance currently exist, yet (b) the management technology is not being applied in the vast majority of residential settings, and particularly not being applied in those staff performance areas that are vital to preventing and/or treating aberrant client behavior (Reid & Schepis, 1986). Consequently, although continued research on the refinement and expansion of existing staff management technology is needed, a more primary research need at this point is to determine how to disseminate the management technology that does exist in regard to assisting managers in typical residential settings to use the supervisory procedures. Such research must focus on how to train managers in the use of organizational behavior management procedures and to maintain their use of the procedures over time. In order to accomplish the latter task, it will most likely be necessary to investigate and disseminate methods of training upper level managers within organizational hierarchies regarding how, in essence, to *manage their managers*. That is, executive staff in residential settings must have the behavioral management skills to ensure that middle management personnel use effective supervisory strategies; senior managers must hold supervisors of direct care staff accountable for direct care staff performance. By ensuring that supervisors of direct service personnel are skilled in and routinely use organizational behavior management strategies, executive personnel can provide their managers with the necessary tools to indeed be accountable.

REFERENCES

Adams, G. L., Tallon, R. J., & Rimell, P. (1980). A comparison of lecture versus role-playing in the training of the use of positive reinforcement. *Journal of Organizational Behavior Management, 2,*(3), 205–212.

Alavosius, M. P., & Sulzer-Azaroff, B. (1986). The effects of performance feedback on the safety of client lifting and transfer. *Journal of Applied Behavior Analysis, 19,* 261–267.

Balcazar, F., Hopkins, B. L., & Suarez, Y. (1986). A critical, objective review of performance feedback. *Journal of Organizational Behavior Management, 7,*(3/4), 65–89.

Bensberg, G. J., & Barnett, C. D. (1966). Attendant training in southern residential facilities for the mentally retarded. Atlanta: Southern Regional Education Board.

Bernstein, G. S., & Karan, O. C. (1978). Preservice training of professionals as behavior managers: A review. *Behavior Therapy, 9,* 124–126.

Bricker, W. A., Morgan, D. G., & Grabowski, J. G. (1972). Development and maintenance of a behavior modification repertoire of cottage attendants through TV feedback. *American Journal of Mental Deficiency, 77,* 128–136.

Brown, K. M., Willis, B. S., & Reid, D. H. (1981). Differential effects of supervisor verbal feedback and feedback plus approval on institutional staff performance. *Journal of Organizational Behavior Management, 3*(1), 57–68.

Burch, M. R., Reiss, M. L., & Bailey, J. S. (1987). A competency-based "hands-on" training package for direct care staff. *Journal of the Association for Persons with Severe Handicaps, 12,* 67–71.

Burg, M. M., Reid, D. H., & Lattimore, J. (1979). Use of a self-recording and supervision program to change institutional staff behavior. *Journal of Applied Behavior Analysis, 12,* 363–375.

Burgio, L. D., Whitman, T. L., & Reid, D. H. (1983). A participative management approach for improving direct-care staff performance in an institutional setting. *Journal of Applied Behavior Analysis, 16,* 37–53.

Christian, W. P. (1983). A case study in the programming and maintenance of institutional change. *Journal of Organizational Behavior Management, 5*(3/4), 99–153.

Dyer, K., Schwartz, I. S., & Luce, S. C. (1984). A supervision program for increasing functional activities for severely handicapped students in a residential setting. *Journal of Applied Behavior Analysis, 17,* 249–259.

Fabry, P. L., & Reid, D. H. (1978). Teaching foster grandparents to train severely handicapped persons. *Journal of Applied Behavior Analysis, 11,* 111–123.

Favell, J. E., Favell, J. E., Riddle, J. I., & Risley, T. R. (1984). Promoting change in mental retardation facilities: Getting services from the paper to the people. In W. P. Christian, G. T. Hannah, & T. J. Glahn (Eds.), *Programming effective human services: Strategies for institutional change and client transition* (pp. 15–37). New York: Plenum.

Faw, G. D., Reid, D. H., Schepis, M. M., Fitzgerald, J. R., & Welty, P. A. (1981). Involving institutional staff in the development and maintenance of sign language skills with profoundly retarded persons. *Journal of Applied Behavior Analysis, 14,* 411–423.

Fielding, L. T., Erricksen, E., & Bettin, B. (1971). Modification of staff behavior: A brief note. *Behavior Therapy, 2,* 550–553.

Fitzgerald, J. R., Reid, D. H., Schepis, M. M., Faw, G. D., Welty, P. A., & Pyfer, L. M. (1984). A rapid training procedure for teaching manual sign language skills to multidisciplinary institutional staff. *Applied Research in Mental Retardation, 5,* 451–469.

Ford, J. E. (1980). A classification system for feedback procedures. *Journal of Organizational Behavior Management, 2*(3), 183–191.

Ford, J. E. (1983). Application of a personalized system of instruction to a large, personnel training program. *Journal of Organizational Behavior Management, 5*(3/4), 57–65.

Fox, D. K., Hopkins, B. L., & Anger, W. K. (1987). The long-term effects of a token economy on safety performance in open-pit mining. *Journal of Applied Behavior Analysis, 20,* 215–224.

Fredericksen, L. W. (1984). Discussion—"If it's not implemented, it can't work." *Journal of Organizational Behavior Management, 6,* 45–52.

Gardner, J. M. (1972). Teaching behavior modification to nonprofessionals. *Journal of Applied Behavior Analysis, 5*, 517–521.

Gardner, J. M. (1973). Training the trainers. A review of research on teaching behavior modification. In R. D. Rubin, J. P. Brady, & J. D. Henderson (Eds.), *Advances in behavior therapy* (Vol. 4). New York: Academic Press.

Gladstone, B. W., & Spencer, C. J. (1977). The effects of modelling on the contingent praise of mental retardation counsellors. *Journal of Applied Behavior Analysis, 10*, 75–84.

Greene, B. F., Willis, B. S., Levy, R., & Bailey, J. S. (1978). Measuring client gains from staff-implemented programs. *Journal of Applied Behavior Analysis, 11*, 395–412.

Hagen, R. L., Craighead, W. E., & Paul, G. L. (1975). Staff reactivity to evaluative behavioral observations. *Behavior Therapy, 6*, 201–205.

Hollander, M. A., & Plutchik, R. (1972). A reinforcement program for psychiatric attendants. *Journal of Behavior Therapy and Experimental Psychiatry, 3*, 297–300.

Hollander, M., Plutchik, R., & Horner, V. (1973). Interaction of patient and attendant reinforcement programs: The "piggyback" effect. *Journal of Consulting and Clinical Psychology, 41*, 43–47.

Horner, R. D. (1980). The effects of an environmental "enrichment" program on the behavior of institutionalized profoundly retarded children. *Journal of Applied Behavior Analysis, 13*, 473–491.

Hutchison, J. M., Jarman, P. H., & Bailey, J. S. (1980). Public posting with a habilitation team: Effects on attendance and performance. *Behavior Modification, 4*, 57–70.

Ivancic, M. T., Reid, D. H., Iwata, B. A., Faw, G. D., & Page, T. J. (1981). Evaluating a supervision program for developing and maintaining therapeutic staff-resident interactions during institutional care routines. *Journal of Applied Behavior Analysis, 14*, 95–107.

Iwata, B. A., Bailey, J. S., Brown, K. M., Foshee, T. J., & Alpern, M. (1976). A performance-based lottery to improve residential care and training by institutional staff. *Journal of Applied Behavior Analysis, 9*, 417–431.

Katz, R. C., & Lutzker, J. R. (1980). A comparison of three methods for training timeout. *Behavior Research of Severe Developmental Disabilities, 1*, 123–130.

Kissel, R. C., Whitman, T. L., & Reid, D. H. (1983). An institutional staff training and self-management program for developing multiple self-care skills in severely/profoundly retarded individuals. *Journal of Applied Behavior Analysis, 16*, 395–415.

Korabek, C. A., Reid, D. H., & Ivancic, M. T. (1981). Improving needed food intake of profoundly handicapped children through effective supervision of institutional staff performance. *Applied Research in Mental Retardation, 2*, 69–88.

Kreitner, R., Reif, W. E., & Morris, M. (1977). Measuring the impact of feedback on the performance of mental health technicians. *Journal of Organizational Behavior Management, 1*, 105–109.

Kunz, G. G. R., Lutzker, J. R., Cuvo, A. J., Eddleman, J., Lutzker, S. Z., Megson, D., & Gulley, B. (1982). Evaluating strategies to improve careprovider performance on health and developmental tasks in an infant care facility. *Journal of Applied Behavior Analysis, 15*, 521–531.

Lattimore, J., Stephens, T. E., Favell, J. E., & Risley, T. R. (1984). Increasing direct care staff compliance to individualized physical therapy body positioning prescriptions: Prescriptive checklists. *Mental Retardation, 22*, 79–84.

Mayhew, G. L., Enyart, P., & Cone, J. D. (1979). Approaches to employee management: Policies and preferences. *Journal of Organizational Behavior Management, 2*, 103–111.

Mansdorf, I. J., & Burstein, Y. (1986). Case manager: A clinical tool for training residential treatment staff. *Behavioral Residential Treatment, 1*, 155–167.

Miller, R., & Lewin, L. M. (1980). Training and management of the psychiatric aide: A critical review. *Journal of Organizational Behavior Management, 2*(4), 295–315.

Montegar, C. A., Reid, D. H., Madsen, C. H., & Ewell, M. D. (1977). Increasing institutional staff-to-resident interactions through inservice training and supervisor approval. *Behavior Therapy, 8*, 533–540.

Page, T. J., Christian, J. G., Iwata, B. A., Reid, D. H., Crow, R. E., & Dorsey, M. F. (1981). Evaluating and training interdisciplinary teams in writing IPP goals and objectives. *Mental Retardation, 19*, 25–27.

Page, T. J., Iwata, B. A., & Reid, D. H. (1982). Pyramidal training: A large-scale application with institutional staff. *Journal of Applied Behavior Analysis, 15*, 335–351.

Panyan, M., Boozer, H., & Morris, N. (1970). Feedback to attendants as a reinforcer for applying operant techniques. *Journal of Applied Behavior Analysis, 3*, 1–4.

Parsons, M. B., Schepis, M. M., Reid, D. H., McCarn, J. E., & Green, C. W. (1987). Expanding the impact of behavioral staff management: A large-scale, long-term application in schools serving severely handicapped students. *Journal of Applied Behavior Analysis, 20*, 139–150.

Pomerleau, O. F., Bobrove, P. H., & Smith, R. H. (1973). Rewarding psychiatric aides for the behavioral improvement of assigned patients. *Journal of Applied Behavior Analysis, 6*, 383–390.

Pommer, D. A., & Streedbeck, D. (1974). Motivating staff performance in an operant learning program for children. *Journal of Applied Behavior Analysis, 7*, 217–221.

Prue, D. M., Krapfl, J. E., Noah, J. C., Cannon, S., & Maley, R. F. (1980). Managing the treatment activities of state hospital staff. *Journal of Organizational Behavior Management, 2*(3), 165–181.

Quilitch, H. R. (1975). A comparison of three staff-management procedures. *Journal of Applied Behavior Analysis, 8*, 59–66.

Quilitch, H. R. (1978). Using a simple feedback procedure to reinforce the submission of written suggestions by mental health employees. *Journal of Organizational Behavior Management, 1*(2), 155–163.

Quilitch, H. R., de Longchamps, G. D., Warden, R. A., & Szczepaniak, C. J. (1977). The effects of announced health inspections upon employee cleaning performance. *Journal of Organizational Behavior Management, 1*(1), 79–88.

Realon, R. E., Wheeler, A. J., Spring, B., & Springer, M. (1986). Evaluating the quality of training delivered by direct care staff in a state mental retardation center. *Behavioral Residential Treatment, 3*, 199–211.

Reid, D. H., & Green, C. W. (in press). Staff training. In J. L. Matson (Ed.), *Handbook of behavior modification for persons with mental retardation* (2nd Edition). New York: Plenum Press.

Reid, D. H., Parsons, M. B., McCarn, J. E., Green, C. W., Phillips, J. F., & Schepis, M. M. (1985). Providing a more appropriate education for severely handicapped persons: Increasing and validating functional classroom tasks. *Journal of Applied Behavior Analysis, 18*, 289–301.

Reid, D. H., & Schepis, M. M. (1986). Direct care staff training. In R. P. Barrett (Ed.), *Severe behavior disorders in the mentally retarded: Nondrug approaches to treatment* (pp. 297–322). New York: Plenum Press.

Reid, D. H., Schuh-Wear, C. L., & Brannon, M. E. (1978). Use of a group contingency to decrease staff absenteeism in a state institution. *Behavior Modification, 2*, 251–266.

Reid, D. H., & Shoemaker, J. (1984). Behavioral supervision: Methods of improving institutional staff performance. In W. P. Christian, G. T. Hannah, & T. J. Glahn (Eds.), *Programming effective human services: Strategies for institutional change and client transition* (pp. 39–61). New York: Plenum Press.

Reid, D. H., & Whitman, T. L. (1983). Behavioral staff management in institutions: A critical review of effectiveness and acceptability. *Analysis and Intervention in Developmental Disabilities, 3*, 131–149.

Repp, A. C., & Barton, L. E. (1980). Naturalistic observations of institutionalized retarded persons: A comparison of licensure decisions and behavioral observations. *Journal of Applied Behavior Analysis, 13*, 333–341.

Repp, A. C., & Deitz, D. E. D. (1978). On the selective use of punishment—suggested guidelines for administrators. *Mental Retardation, 16*, 250–254.

Repp, A. C., & Deitz, D. E. D. (1979). Improving administrative-related staff behaviors at a state institution. *Mental Retardation, 17*, 185–192.

Seys, D. M., & Duker, P. C. (1978). Improving residential care for the retarded by differential reinforcement of high rates of ward-staff behaviour. *Behavioural Analysis and Modification, 2*, 203–210.

Seys, D. M., & Duker, P. C. (1986). Effects of a supervisory treatment package on staff-mentally retarded resident interactions. *American Journal of Mental Deficiency, 90*, 388–394.

Shoemaker, J., & Reid, D. H. (1980). Decreasing chronic absenteeism among institutional staff: Effects of a low-cost attendance program. *Journal of Organizational Behavior Management, 2,*(4), 317–328.

Smith, D. W., & Wells, M. E. (1983). Use of a microcomputer to assist staff in documenting resident progress. *Mental Retardation, 21,* 111–115.

Sneed, T. J., & Bible, G. H. (1979). An administrative procedure for improving staff performance in an institutional setting for retarded persons. *Mental Retardation, 17,* 92–94.

Spangler, P. F., & Marshall, A. M. (1983). The unit play manager as a facilitator of purposeful activities among institutionalized profoundly and severely retarded boys. *Journal of Applied Behavior Analysis, 16,* 345–349.

Stoddard, L. T., McIlvane, W. J., McDonagh, E. C., & Kledaras, J. B. (1986). The use of picture programs in teaching direct care staff. *Applied Research in Mental Retardation, 7,* 349–358.

Stolz, S. B. (1981). Adoption of innovations from applied behavioral research: "Does anybody care?" *Journal of Applied Behavior Analysis, 14,* 491–505.

van den Pol, R. A., Reid, D. H., & Fuqua, R. W. (1983). Peer training of safety-related skills to institutional staff: Benefits for trainers and trainees. *Journal of Applied Behavior Analysis, 16,* 139–156.

Wallace, C. J., Davis, J. R., Liberman, R. P., & Baker, V. (1973). Modeling and staff behavior. *Journal of Consulting and Clinical Psychology, 41,* 422–425.

Welsch, W. V., Ludwig, C., Radiker, J. E., & Krapfl, J. E. (1973). Effects of feedback on daily completion of behavior modification projects. *Mental Retardation, 11,* 24–26.

Whitman, T. L., Scibak, J. W., & Reid, D. H. (1983). *Behavior modification with the severely and profoundly retarded: Research and application.* New York: Academic Press.

Zlomke, L. C., & Benjamin, Jr., V. A., (1983). Staff inservice: Measuring effectiveness through client behavior change. *Education and Training of the Mentally Retarded, 18,* 125–130.